DATE DUE

MAR 1 1		
MAR 3 1		
MAY 2 9		
JUN 1 6		
SEP 1 5		
SEP 2 9		
NOV 2 6		
OCT 8 '97		

A
TEEN-AGE
GUIDE
TO
HEALTHY
SKIN
and HAIR

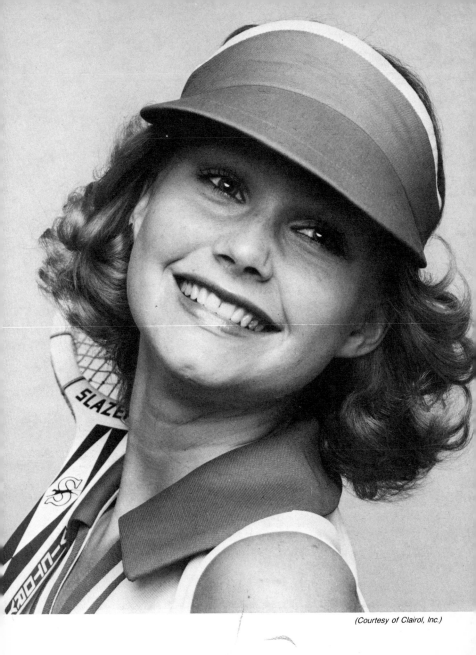

A TEEN-AGE GUIDE TO HEALTHY SKIN and HAIR

THIRD EDITION, REVISED AND UPDATED

Irwin I. Lubowe, M.D., and Barbara Huss

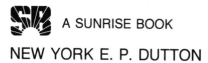 A SUNRISE BOOK

NEW YORK E. P. DUTTON

For information contact: E.P. Dutton, 2 Park Avenue, New York, N.Y. 10016

Library of Congress Catalog Card Number: 73-190375.

ISBN: 0-87690-335-9 (cloth)
       0-87690-334-0 (paper)

Published simultaneously in Canada by Clarke, Irwin & Company Limited, Toronto and Vancouver

Designed by Ernie Haim

10 9 8 7 6 5 4 3 2 1

This book is dedicated to teen-agers everywhere who will make this a better place for living

Books by Irwin I. Lubowe, M.D.

Cosmetics and the Skin *(with Fred V. Wells)*

Tell Me the Truth, Doctor

New Hope for Your Hair

New Hope for Your Skin

Dermatological Formulary and Pharmaceutical Manual *(with Morris Dauer)*

Modern Guide to Skin Care and Beauty

A Teen-Age Guide to Healthy Skin and Hair *(with Barbara Huss)*

CONTENTS

ILLUSTRATIONS

DRAWINGS AND DIAGRAMS

ACKNOWLEDGMENTS

In the preparation and writing of this book, we drew upon Dr. Lubowe's clinical experience gained from active hospital and office practice and upon Miss Huss's experience as a teen-age adviser and writer in the cosmetic and pharmaceutical fields.

We are indebted to Ruth Lubowe for her editorial services and her writing of the glossary. Our appreciative thanks go to Cathi Hunt and Jill Hee of Clairol Inc. for information and helpful suggestions on hair coloring; to home economist Ellen Katz for her advice on nutrition; to Dr. Mitchell Rosenthal and Irwin Simmons of Phoenix House for their assistance in providing information for the chapter on drugs and for permission to quote them freely; to Terry Bellicha of the National Clearinghouse for Alcohol Information for providing a wealth of material on teen-age drinking; and to Gina Johnson of Planned Parenthood for her informative aid.

Our appreciative thanks also go to *Today's Health,* printed by the American Medical Association, for permission to reproduce the illustrations on the anatomy of the skin and effects of ultraviolet light in suntanning of the skin; and to the National Highway Traffic Safety Administration for allowing us to reproduce their table on the relationship of alcohol to safe driving. We also are grateful to the following organizations for permission to use their excellent photographs: *American Hairdresser Salon Owner,* Clairol Inc., the Cleanliness Bureau, the Andrew Jergens Company, *Men's Hairstylist,* Planned Parenthood, Sebring Products Inc.

INTRODUCTION

You are unique.

No one else in the world has a combination of tissues, muscles, skin, hair, brains and emotions like yours. Agreed?

You are unique for many other good reasons. Your body is going through many physical changes as you grow into maturity. Your feelings and emotions are changing. Your relationships with other people are adjusting also. You are forming the attitudes and objectives that will stay with you the rest of your life.

You are unique because, more than ever before in history, you influence others both older and younger than yourself. Your influence in the world, your country and your community is seen in your involvement with important issues. People listen. They respect your ideals and beliefs. You influence our statesmen.

You are unique because you influence music, art, fashion, food, cosmetics and fads and fancies. You, as a young adult, help spend several billion dollars a year on all these things. You affect our whole nation's economy.

The young adult years are turbulent. We believe they can be less so if you understand clearly some important body functions, what can go wrong and how problems can be treated. In this book, while emphasizing the functions, problems and care of your skin and hair, we discuss in detail the related subjects of hairstyling, grooming, cosmetics, diet and weight control, sports and exercise. In this edition, we also tackle the "heavy" but vitally important subjects of drugs and alcohol, contraceptives and venereal disease. We hope you'll use this information to increase your own knowledge and your own healthy good looks.

And we wish you every happiness!

—THE AUTHORS

A
TEEN-AGE
GUIDE
TO
HEALTHY
SKIN
and HAIR

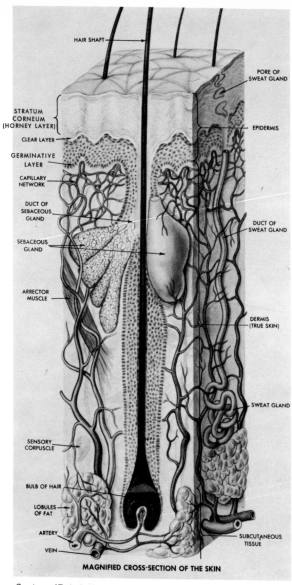

HAIR SHAFT

PORE OF
SWEAT GLAND

STRATUM
CORNEUM
(HORNEY LAYER)

EPIDERMIS

CLEAR LAYER

GERMINATIVE
LAYER

CAPILLARY
NETWORK

DUCT OF
SEBACEOUS
GLAND

DUCT OF
SWEAT GLAND

SEBACEOUS
GLAND

ARRECTOR
MUSCLE

DERMIS
(TRUE SKIN)

SWEAT GLAND

SENSORY
CORPUSCLE

BULB OF HAIR

LOBULES
OF FAT

ARTERY

SUBCUTANEOUS
TISSUE

VEIN

MAGNIFIED CROSS-SECTION OF THE SKIN

Courtesy of Today's Health, *published by the American Medical Association*

CHAPTER ONE
YOUR PRIVATE
SPACE SUIT

> It keeps much that is hostile in our
> surroundings from getting at our
> all-too-vulnerable innards and, at the
> same time, keeps those innards from seeping
> out.
>
> —*Albert Rosenfeld*

Your space suit totals almost twenty-one square feet. It cools you when you're hot and warms you when you're cold. It sends sensations to the brain and muscles, it fights off attacking organisms and it throws off body wastes. It's the largest and one of the most important organs of the body.

We're talking, of course, about your skin—that necessary item that keeps you all together.

What *is* the skin? If you put a microscope to a square inch of skin, what would you see? The top layer of skin is the *stratum corneum*. Its job is to act as a protective armor against heat, sun and external injuries. It varies in thickness in different parts of the body. The most delicate skin is on your eyelids—the toughest, on the soles of your feet and the palms of your hands. Skin can be thicker on some people than on others. Have you ever known a

1

girl with an almost translucent skin, so that the blue veins underneath show clearly? Her skin really is thin, and this has nothing to do with her temper!

Below the *stratum corneum* is the *stratum lucidum,* a clear layer. Next comes the *stratum granulosum,* a granular layer, and the *stratum germinativum,* the prickle cell layer. The bottom layer is the basal cell layer. Each of these skin layers is in a continuous process of movement. As the cells of the outer layer become hard and lose their nuclei, they are cast off and replaced by new, active cells that migrate upward. This process of cell movement and change is called *keratinization,* and usually takes about twenty-five days.

The skin layers have important work to do. They contain sebaceous glands that manufacture an oil that lubricates the skin and hair. They contain your body's sweat glands and hair shafts (follicles). They house the busy blood and lymph vessels, the nerve-ending cells, muscles, fat and connective tissue elements.

It seems hard to believe, but just one square inch of skin contains:

78 nerves
650 sweat glands
19 or 20 blood vessels
78 sensory apparatuses for heat
13 sensory apparatuses for cold
1,300 nerve endings to record pain
19,500 sensory cells at the ends of nerve fibers
160 to 165 pressure apparatuses for the sense of touch
95 to 100 sebaceous glands
65 hairs and muscles
19,500,000 cells

If you are a whiz at math, you can multiply all those components in one square inch of skin and get a pretty fantastic figure for all twenty-one square feet of you!

Among the functions the skin performs, one of the most fascinating is *pigmentation,* or the coloring of the skin itself. Development of pigment occurs in the basal cell layer of the skin. Here,

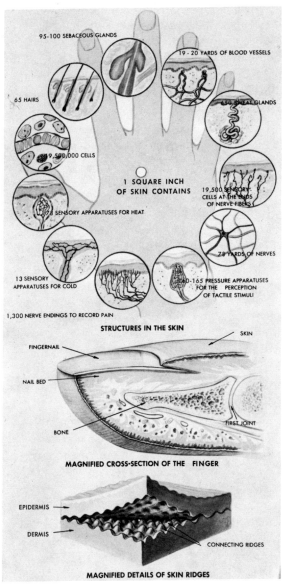

95-100 SEBACEOUS GLANDS

19 - 20 YARDS OF BLOOD VESSELS

65 HAIRS

650 SWEAT GLANDS

9,500,000 CELLS

1 SQUARE INCH
OF SKIN CONTAINS

19,500 SENSORY
CELLS AT THE ENDS
OF NERVE FIBERS

8 SENSORY APPARATUSES FOR HEAT

7-8 YARDS OF NERVES

13 SENSORY
APPARATUSES FOR COLD

160-165 PRESSURE APPARATUSES
FOR THE   PERCEPTION
OF TACTILE STIMULI

1,300 NERVE ENDINGS TO RECORD PAIN

STRUCTURES IN THE SKIN

SKIN

FINGERNAIL

NAIL BED

FIRST JOINT

BONE

MAGNIFIED CROSS-SECTION OF THE   FINGER

EPIDERMIS

DERMIS

CONNECTING RIDGES

MAGNIFIED DETAILS OF SKIN RIDGES

Courtesy of Today's Health, *published by the American Medical Association*

cells convert an amino acid into the skin coloring pigment, *melanin.*

Melanin is the ingredient that gives the races of mankind their different skin tones. The pale skin of the Caucasian, the reddish tint of the Indian, the golden tone of the Oriental and the brownish-black coloring of the full-blooded Black are all determined by the amount of melanin in the skin.

When a human being or an animal lacks essential pigment, he is called an *albino.* His skin and eyes have a pinkish tinge, which actually comes from the red blood circulating beneath his "no color" skin and eyes. Albinism is hereditary, but it is not disabling. Except for being careful about exposure to the sun, an albino can lead a normal life. (It's interesting, in reading ancient history and mythology, to realize that early peoples often worshiped albinos, believing them to be special deities.)

But back to the skin. It also protects, by covering your bones, muscles, arteries, nerves and tissues. Lying loosely like a sheet upon a mattress of muscle, the skin bears the brunt of irritation, absorbs shock and protects essential internal organs from harm. The skin's surface also shields you from harmful gases and alkalies which could upset the chemical composition of the blood.

The skin is your body's thermostat, too. Inside your body, your blood temperature is about one degree higher than 98.6 degrees. In very hot weather, when the air temperature is about as hot as your blood temperature, the skin carries off the body heat in the form of perspiration. When the weather is cold, blood vessels under the skin constrict, keeping body heat inside to warm you. Efficient, isn't it?

Far more complicated than the best electronic brain invented by man, the skin is a busy message center, telegraphing sensations of heat, cold, pain and danger. The messages sent by the nerve endings move fast, whizzing to the brain and then to the muscles, which react by reflex action.

How fast the nerve endings operate is proved when you touch a hot potato. The message goes like this: "Hot! Ouch!

Hands off!'' And in a split second, your brain receives the message and your muscles move your fingers away fast. Under danger, the skin also reacts. Those old clichés that advertise horror movies—"makes your flesh creep," "gives you goose pimples," "hair-raising"—are all based on truth. When you are frightened or in danger, your hair muscles suddenly constrict, raising goose pimples on your skin, or creating the sensation that your skin is crawling. Your hair actually can stand on end when the skin muscles contract, pushing the hair outward. If you've ever watched a cat's fur bristle at the sight of danger or an enemy, you've seen this principle in action.

Meanwhile, deep in the skin, its vast manufacturing process is busily turning out *sebum,* which is deposited on the epidermis. Sebum is a lubricant—your body's own brand of cold cream. Too much or too little sebum can cause oily or dry skin. Acne and dandruff also are caused by trouble in the sebaceous glands. Perspiration is another excretion of the skin. Your sweat ducts give off one to two quarts a day, according to the temperature. You also perspire more when you are exercising heavily, or are tense and under stress.

We've mentioned just some of the skin's many jobs. You also should know that the skin "breathes" through millions of pores, absorbing oxygen and certain other substances, giving off carbon dioxide. This carbon dioxide combines with the perspiration and amino acids of your skin to form an "acid mantle" on the surface. The acid mantle helps ward off bacterial infection. When it is disrupted by alkaline soaps or detergents, skin rashes and dishpan hands may often result.

Whether you're sprawled on a sofa watching television, skiing down a snowy slope, "sweating out" an exam or just plain sleeping, your skin is always working to keep you active and healthy.

But sometimes, something goes wrong. What happens? How can you correct it?

CHAPTER TWO
ACNE: THE TEEN-AGE PROBLEM

Most teen-agers—over 80 percent of you—suffer from acne. More males get acne than females, but it's equally distressing to both sexes. Sometimes described as the price of maturing, acne is a disturbance of the sebaceous glands which results in a crop of bumps, pimples, blackheads and, sometimes, ugly scars. Acne is certainly not fatal, but it probably causes more anguish than any other health problem.

But don't despair; we have good news for you! Within just the last couple of years, new therapy has been developed that is highly effective against this enemy of adolescence. (In fact, for this new edition, we've scrapped everything we had written before on the subject.)

Just the other day Tim, a fifteen-year-old, came into the office. His face was pitted and scarred with acne lesions. He seemed withdrawn, moody and depressed.

"My mother insisted on setting up this appointment for me," he said. "But there's probably nothing you can do. It's something I'll just have to live with."

He was wrong. There's a lot we can do. Delay just makes matters worse. If only more of you and your parents realized that acne can—and should—be treated promptly by a physician!

6

Treatment can prevent so many miserable moments. It can restore self-confidence and good looks. It can prevent a pitted or pockmarked face. And it can also remove the evidence of acne scars. This case had a happy ending. We were able, through a course of treatment, to prevent new outbreaks of the disease and to remove the scars. Tim literally felt and looked like a new person.

WHY IT HAPPENS

Acne primarily occurs in adolescence because these are the years when your body is busily secreting the male (androgen) hormones and the female (estrogen) hormones, but in different proportions for each sex. When your body's balance of androgen-estrogen hormones goes out of whack, so do the sebaceous glands of the *dermis,* or deep skin.

Overactivity of the sebaceous glands of the dermis causes extra amounts of sebum, the skin lubricant, to rise to the skin surface. The sebum, like a layer of cold cream, makes the skin surface oily and encourages the growth of bacteria. The sebum

FORMATION OF PIMPLES

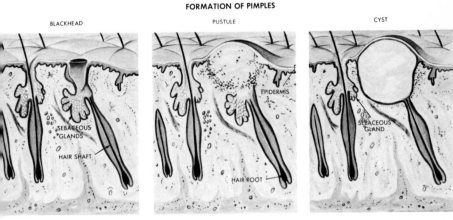

Courtesy of Today's Health, *published by the American Medical Association*

also plugs up the pores of the skin. These plugged-up pores result in *milia* (whiteheads) or *comedones* (blackheads). The difference between them, incidentally, is that the blackheads have their ends exposed to the air, and become oxidized and darkened by sulfur deposition.

If the sebum has no way of exiting from the skin, it stays below the skin surface in the follicle and causes a raised red bump (papule or pimple) that becomes infected. To fight the infection, your white corpuscles enter the fray. Some of these cause formation of pus. It is these pus-filled, infectious lesions that are the most disturbing form of acne. And, if untreated, they become the source of ugly pitting and scarring.

In teen-age males, the worst bouts of acne occur just after their bodies start producing excessive amounts of a male hormone, testosterone. In young women, acne outbreaks occur at the beginning of each menstrual period, when estrogen hormone production goes down and causes an imbalance.

While hormone imbalance is the major cause of acne, there are others that you should know about. Emotional upheavals cause skin upheavals. Tensions, temper, relationships with others, worry—all contribute to the problem. Here are some typical examples from our files:

"My skin troubles started about a year ago, when my parents and I didn't seem to be tuned in at all. We fought constantly. *They* fought constantly. Now my parents are divorced, and my skin has been haywire ever since."

"I'm a new girl in town, Doctor, and moving to a big city from a New England village is like coming to another planet! I miss my friends back home, I'm having a hard time in school, and just look at my face."

"I'd been going with a girl who really meant a lot to me. Then four months ago, she broke up with me. When she broke up, my face broke out! Now I feel so self-conscious about my looks that I can't bring myself to date anyone."

Each of these problems triggered skin trouble. For you see,

it's not just the hormones that are changing in your body, it's your physiology and sympathetic nervous system, too. We now believe that emotional intensity stimulates the sebaceous glands to produce more oil and hence, more acne.

Too many fats in your diet are a common cause of acne. Since the sebaceous glands need food to function, they draw upon the daily intake of food that is transported to the skin by the blood. The worst villains are fatty meats, carbohydrates, chocolate, cocoa, spices, iodized salt and shellfish. Those who are acne-prone should either avoid these foods altogether, or eat them infrequently.

Faulty digestion of the food you eat also contributes to acne. You remember that one of the skin's functions is to excrete waste. If the bowels are not functioning properly, more of a strain is put upon the skin's excretion efforts. Fresh fruit, vegetables and bulk in the diet are "musts" to keep digestion and waste elimination performing efficiently.

Bacteria breeding anywhere in the body can add to the spread of acne. An infection of the tonsils, appendix, lymph nodes, teeth or gums can encourage acne. This can be treated quickly by a doctor if you don't ignore the warning symptoms.

We also know that acne may be hereditary. If your father or mother ever had a severe case of acne, you may very well have the same tendency. Today, of course, we can deal with it much more effectively.

Sloppy personal hygiene, especially of the hair and scalp, causes dandruff and oil to spill onto the face, creating acne on the forehead.

In some female patients, use of the Pill causes cystic acne. For them, we recommend other methods of birth control.

Another cause of acne is the combination of hot weather and high humidity. This "sweat acne" is usually found on the forehead, and we'll talk about a treatment for it later on.

WHAT CAN BE DONE ABOUT IT

Now let's look at the bright side. There is a new antibiotic treatment that has revolutionized the handling and treatment of acne! Antibiotic therapy is not new, of course. For a number of years we have known that antibiotics are the most effective approach in the treatment of all types of acne. Past measures have included prescribing two capsules daily of tetracycline, erythromycin, vibramycin, or one of the other "mycins." These antibiotics work to suppress the formation of unsaturated fatty acids, which produce the acne lesions. There have been some drawbacks, however. The capsules are expensive, and antibiotics taken internally can cause nausea, diarrhea and vaginitis in some.

The new antibiotic treatment comes in less expensive lotion form, applied directly onto the affected skin surface. Since it is not taken by mouth and swallowed into the system, it causes no internal side effects. And there have not been any reported cases of skin irritation caused by use of the lotion. (It must be kept refrigerated, however, to maintain its therapeutic effect.)

One note about antibiotics: we advise patients who are using antibiotics to take four ounces of fat-free yogurt daily. The yogurt keeps the intestinal tract functioning smoothly, and prevents decrease of certain necessary normal bacteria in the intestine which antibiotics diminish. Yogurt is one of the few "fast foods" that really is good for you, in more ways than one!

Another effective form of treatment used by skin specialists is vitamin A, which aids the normal functioning of the skin and prevents the formation of blackheads. This comes in tablet, swab, liquid or cream form. It must be prescribed by a doctor, since it does have some side effects and certain precautions must be taken during its use.

SEVEN SIMPLE STEPS

Time to turn to other forms of treatment. You can control acne by:

1. Cleaning the skin. It is absolutely vital to remove oil, grease and air pollutants from the surface of the skin. Bacteria breed in oil. They, in turn, cause infection of the acne cysts. Thorough cleansing means several face washings a day, careful rinsing and drying. If you tend at all to acne, then use an antiseptic soap, such as Safeguard, Dial, Zest, Bonne Bell 10-06, or pHiso-Hex. Other antiseptic soaps your doctor may recommend are those that have keratolytic action, stripping off oils from the skin surface. These include such products as Acne Aid, Sastid, Foxtex and Proseca.

The use of abrasive products is suggested in some cases. These not only clean, but loosen blackheads and the upper layer of the corneum. These come in the form of soaps (Pernox, Brasivol, Persadox) and as gels (Transact, Xerac, Benzagel).

One problem that acne creates is the forming of pus-filled skin lesions, which must be dried out. There are a number of medicated lotions that your doctor can recommend to dry these up on the face, chest and back. They contain sulfur, salicylic acid, resorcinol, antiseptics, benzoyl peroxide and other "degreasing" agents. If areas of the face are reddened and swollen, they can be treated with compresses of boric acid and of Burow's solution applied directly to the affected area.

Obviously, cosmetics should be used with care. Don't use greasy products, foundations and creams. One of the basic problems of acne is too much grease (sebum is your skin's own cold cream, remember?) and you don't want to add more grease to a skin already saturated with it. If you tend to have a very oily complexion, also use an astringent several times a week to clean and dry up the skin surface. These contain alcohol, acetone and witch hazel, and work by reducing the amount of oil secretions on the skin surface.

2. Cleaning the hair and scalp. As you've already seen, greasy hair and dandruff are a major cause of acne, particularly on the forehead. For most people, a mild neutral soap or detergent shampoo should do the trick. If you have any dandruff problems, then use an antidandruff shampoo at least twice a week. One of the most effective ingredients in these is zinc pyrithione, which has no toxic reactions. It is found in Head and Shoulders, Breck

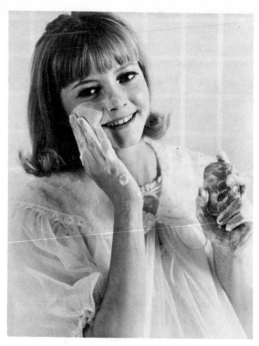

You can help control acne by keeping your skin scrupulously clean. The facial illustrated here is an effective means of removing bacteria, grease and oil as they accumulate on the skin surface. Using an antiseptic soap, work up a rich lather of suds, stroking gently upward from the chin. Then stroke across the cheekbones from the bridge of the nose outward to the temples. With lather and fingertips, use a circular motion to clean around mouth area and a stroking motion on the forehead between the eyes. Let soapsuds set on your face while you lather neckline and throat area thoroughly. Complete the facial by rinsing first with warm water, then with cool water, and pat dry. *(Andrew Jergens Company Photo)*

Formula 1 and Zincon shampoos. Other effective antidandruff shampoos are Selsun Blue and Dawex.

While you're at it, avoid hair-grooming products that are greasy or sticky. They just add to production of oils on the scalp, and many cases of facial acne don't improve until all sources of oil, grease and dandruff on the scalp have been removed.

3. Keeping your hands off your face. Squeezing pimples or picking at your face is a surefire way to spread infection under the skin surface, causing a larger crop of nasty-looking bumps. Go to your doctor for treatment. He can remove the blackheads and whiteheads, incising each pustule with a special instrument. Then he cleans out the pus, cleanses the skin surface and applies an astringent to close the incision. When done by a doctor, this method avoids scarring, which can result if you "do-it-yourself."

4. Avoiding patent medicine "cures." Most mail-order miracles are worthless, and a waste of money. Always check with your doctor and let him prescribe what's best for you and your own skin. As you have seen, there really is an army of effective acne fighters available today, so why take a chance?

5. Eating and exercising intelligently. If a certain food seems to make you break out, don't eat it. Refer back to that list of acne-causing foods on page 9. And while experts now agree that a special acne diet is not absolutely necessary, they do agree that a diet that covers the basic four food groups is good for everyone, and especially good for acne-prone people. (For more details, see Chapter XVI, Food for Thought.)

Combining good eating habits with generous daily helpings of exercise keeps the brain and body fit. Fatigue, sluggishness and "televisionitis" are danger symptoms of dull health and dull, acne-prone skin. Exercise is "in" for everyone these days; do make sure you read Chapter XV.

6. Sunning sensibly. While scientists know that some exposure to sunlight, or to the ultraviolet rays of the sun lamp, is beneficial for those with acne, there are some dangers you should know about. One is so obvious that we shouldn't have to mention it. We will anyway, just because it happens so often. The danger is severe sunburn, caused by too long a session under the sun lamp, or out in the broiling sun.

One form of acne, "sweat acne," appears when hot sun and high humidity combine to cause breakouts on the forehead. Dermatan, a new suntan lotion or gel that contains an antiperspirant, appears to be a promising treatment for this. It reduces the acne while promoting a nice golden tan.

7. Playing it cool. Physically and emotionally, the teen-age years are those of extraordinary change. Naturally, the nervous energy you spend on worry contributes to the state of your health and your skin. Intense emotions stimulate the sebaceous glands to produce more oil and, correspondingly, more acne. In some cases, your doctor may feel it necessary to prescribe a mild sedative or tranquilizer to help preserve your "cool" and your complexion. But as more and more evidence piles up indicating the dangers of *dependency upon any drug,* many doctors prefer their patients not to travel that route at all. (Valium, a widely prescribed tranquilizer, is now proved to have highly unpleasant withdrawal symptoms when its use is ceased.)

So the best course is to try to be philosophical about the changes you are experiencing. Centuries ago, it was said in the Bible that "This, too, shall pass." It's just as true today as when it was written.

TREATMENT FOR SERIOUS SCARS

Sad to say, some young people suffer from severe, infectious acne which has left disfiguring scars and lesions. However, there is hope for them. There are three procedures used today which can remove the scars and help restore normal good looks.

1. Dermabrasion is one method often performed in the skin specialist's office. The face is "frozen" by means of a chemical spray that leaves the skin surface insensitive and stiff. A motor-driven brush is then run gently over the face, planing away the excessive irregular scar tissue. After the planing, a crust forms, which lasts for about a week. The face will remain reddened for several weeks, and should not be exposed to the ultraviolet rays of the sun or to a sun lamp for that period.

2. Peeling is another procedure performed by a skin specialist. It is used to help correct shallow acne pits. The doctor applies a mild acid solution to the skin, which has the effect of whitening the skin and reducing the depth of the scar. In this process, the chemical reaches only the top layer of the skin, and in a few days the face starts to peel. Usually it takes from seven to ten days for the "peeled" skin to slough off all the unwanted tissue and replace it with fresh tissue.

3. Chemotherapy is a third procedure that is used in more serious cases where scarring is deeper. It is similar to peeling, except that trichloroacetic acid is used, which is a stronger solution than the compounds used in simple peeling. The acid is applied by the doctor with a cotton applicator, and the peeling is complete in two to three weeks.

No method of treatment will cure acne overnight. Sometimes, when your general health is not up to par, or you get blue or tense, you may have a setback or two. But you mustn't get discouraged! It takes time to build up the body's immunity, and to calm overactive sebaceous glands.

In the meantime, there is more hope for acne sufferers than ever before. And your own good sense will tell you that prompt treatment can make the face that faces the future a happy one!

CHAPTER THREE
ONE EXTREME TO THE OTHER

Nancy's skin is oily. Her older sister, Anne, has dry skin. Their mother has sensitive skin. Is skin type a matter of age? Or of sex? Or of where you live?

All of these factors are related. We know that both males and females tend toward oily skins in the teen years. The sebaceous glands that produce the skin lubricant, sebum, are especially active in adolescence due to hormones sending a new supply of oil to the skin surface about every three hours. And, as we've said in the last chapter, oiliness encourages enlarged pores, blemishes and acne.

Where you live, and the amount of time you spend outdoors, also affect your skin. Cold, dry or windy climates tend to dry out the skin, while humid weather stimulates the production of oil.

To determine your own skin type, rub a piece of a brown paper bag over your face when you get up in the morning. If the paper turns transparent, you have oily skin; if only a slight stain appears, then your skin is normal; if the paper doesn't change texture or color at all, then your skin is dry. Let's look at the specific ways of caring for different skin types.

Oiliness occurs most often in adolescence. To keep a com-

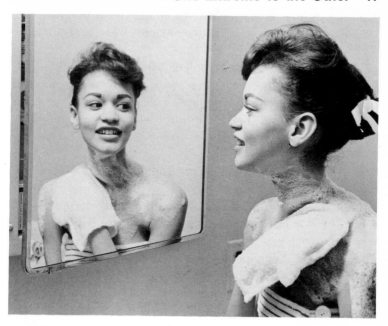

Girls with oily skins should pay special attention to neckline and shoulders, where blemishes may breed. For a smooth, pretty neck and shoulders, massage suds into the area with a bath mitt or bath brush. *(Cleanliness Bureau Photo)*

plexion clear and blemish-free, it's important to remove the oils that rise regularly to the skin surface like clockwork. Therefore, be scrupulous about washing your face and neck at least two to three times a day, using an antiseptic soap or detergent cleanser. When lathering, pay special attention to the center strip of your forehead, nose and chin, since it contains the largest number of oil-producing glands. Complete your cleansing routine by rinsing carefully with lukewarm water, followed by a tingling splash of cold water or an astringent. Then pat dry.

Useful aids for oily skin types are the alcohol-saturated pads such as Sebanil Towelettes that are kept moist in foil packets. Tuck several in your pocket or purse and use them for quick cleansing during the day. Witch hazel and cleansing grains are other aids that temporarily tighten enlarged pores and stimulate circulation.

If oiliness is a serious problem, ask your doctor about the liquid cleansers that contain detergent, sulfur or salicylic acid. You apply these to the face and neck with a cotton pad, changing pads until no trace of grease or grime is left. Males with oily skins should use an alcohol-based aftershave regularly to help remove those surface oils.

Young women with oily skins should be particularly careful about using makeup. Avoid oily, greasy preparations. Instead, use liquid oil-free foundations that are slightly drying. Never apply a new "paint job" over one that is several hours old, and always remove every trace of makeup when cleansing your face at night. Do make it a point to scrub neck and shoulders, where blemishes are apt to breed. Use a bath mitt or brush to scrub suds into those areas and rinse off well.

Oily skins usually mean oily scalps and hair. Shampoo several times a week or about every four days, using a soap or detergent shampoo. *Grease* to the contrary, don't use oily or sticky hair preparations.

The way you style your hair is important, too. An attractive fifteen-year-old whom we helped with an excessively oily skin found that by wearing her hair shorter and away from her forehead, she could wash and set it more easily. And by keeping bangs off her forehead, she did not aggravate the oily forehead condition. Instead of setting lotions and sprays, both sexes benefit from blow dryers if they have oily skins and scalps.

The foods you eat can affect an oily skin condition. Foods containing lots of iodine (shellfish, peanuts, saltwater fish) and too many greasy, fatty foods can contribute to an oversupply of sebum. Foods with vitamin A, often called the complexion vitamin, are known to keep skin, eyes, glands and membranes healthy. While it is found in fatty foods, which you want to avoid, it's also present in leafy vegetables, yellow vegetables, fruits, liver, eggs and fortified margarine.

An oily skin may stay with you all your life or it may become drier when you reach your twenties or thirties. Kept under control, an oily skin can be nice to have. It keeps a glow of youth and an elasticity longer than other types. It can take severe temperature changes without roughening or chapping. And it tans easily.

What about the other extreme—dry skin? It may surprise you, but a recent survey showed that three out of every five adult women suffer from dry skin. It is the most common complexion problem in America.

What causes it? Climate is one culprit. The violent temperature changes from winter to summer, the extremes of indoor heat and air conditioning, all contribute to dry skin. Another cause of dry skin is that the sebaceous glands do not manufacture enough lubrication for the skin, so that it flakes and dries, is subject to sunburning and chapping and tends to develop tiny lines. In other cases, the acid mantle of the skin, which helps destroy bacteria on the skin surface, is removed through continuous use of alkalies or harsh soaps, leaving the skin sensitive to irritation.

In our medical practice we have encountered a condition for which we have coined the name "city skin"—the drying, flaking and reddened skin of the city dweller who comes in contact with noxious industrial and other air pollutants. Your doctor may prescribe specially formulated creams for this condition.

In general, all dry skins must be nourished with a balance of emollients and oils. These soften the surface and help prevent the skin's natural moisture from escaping into the air. This process of nourishing dry skin is called *hydrating.* There are many moisturizing products formulated especially for dry skins, and they should be used daily after cleansing. Some brand names are Germaine Monteil's Super Moist, Visible Difference by Elizabeth Arden, Almay's Moisturizer, and Estée Lauder's special moisturizer, Bonne Bell Moisture Cream.

As for cleansing dry skin, you should take special precautions. In the morning, wash with warm water and a nonalkaline complexion bar or a creamy skin cleanser, lotion or cleansing cream, such as Pond's Light Whipped Cold Cream, Neutrogena

Dry-Skin Soap, Basis Soap, Oilatum Soap, or Alpha Keri Soap. During the day, freshen up with a bit of cleansing lotion that does not contain alcohol. At night, cleanse gently again and finish with a protective moisturizer.

The skin of the body tends to be much drier than that of the face and neck, even among oily skin types. Relaxing tub-soaks in

Dry skin must be nourished with a balance of oils and other liquids, a process called *hydrating*. An after-bath body lotion is a good way to combat dryness and leave skin silky smooth. And remember, in bathing or showering, don't use very hot or very cold water on your skin. *(Andrew Jergens Company Photo)*

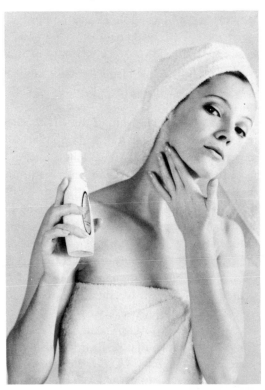

warm water and bath oil will lubricate the skin for several hours. (Just be sure never to use very hot or very cold water on your skin.) Body lotions are helpful, too, especially during the winter months. These include such products as Vaseline Intensive Care Lotion, Johnson's Baby Lotion, Aqua Care-HP Lotion, Keri Lotion and Nivea Lotion.

Cosmetics for dry-skinned girls should be those with creamy formulas. Liquid makeup and pressed-powder-plus-foundation are helpful also. If your skin is extra dry, ask your doctor about the use of hypoallergenic cosmetics.

Dry-skinned males often find their faces feel especially tender and sensitive after shaving. If this is a problem for you, use shave creams with added moisturizers and, after shaving, a non-drying lotion. Or follow up with talcum or baby powder.

Dry-skin types also need plenty of vitamin A. In addition to lean meats, green and yellow vegetables, fruits and eggs, you'll find vitamin A in butter, whole milk, cream cheese and ice cream. If your complexion is clear and your weight is right, you'll want to have these foods regularly in your diet. When someone suffers from extremely dry skin, the doctor may prescribe supplements of vitamin A in capsule form.

Moisture, like oil, rises to the skin surface from deep below it. To keep natural moisture flowing, drink your full quota of water and fruit juices daily.

Dry skin is beautiful when properly managed, since it tends to have a velvet-smooth texture, with small pores and delicate coloration. But it must have regular, tender loving care!

Those of you with normal skins don't have to pamper your complexions as much as those of you who tend to the two extremes. But the basic rules of careful cleansing and rinsing in warm water still apply. Some good cleansers for you are Noxzema Skin Cream and Neutrogena Soap. Your skin will also benefit from the use of a moisturizer and a body lotion.

Many people have what is known as a "combination skin" —that is, a complexion that is basically normal or dry with an oily strip centered down the forehead, nose and chin. Unless the problem is extremely severe and requires special products prescribed by your doctor, you can treat a combination skin with the same routines outlined for normal to dry skins, but by adding the use of an antiseptic cleanser and an astringent on the oiliest portions of the face. Germaine Monteil's new Montage line and Revlon's Formula Z are designed to deal with dryness and oiliness at the same time by moisturizing below the surface and absorbing excess oil on the skin surface superficially.

We will discuss special precautions to take outdoors in Chapters V and XV. But for now, remember that extremes in your life-style also affect your skin. When the face that looks blearily back from your mirror after a bout of late studying or partying is broken out and beat, try to get yourself back on an even keel. A healthy skin requires plenty of sleep and rest to function efficiently.

CHAPTER FOUR
ALLERGIES, ITCHES AND INFECTIONS

Benjamin sneezes
When a cat stalks by,
Benjamin wheezes
When the sun's in the sky,
Benjamin itches
When he drinks tea,
Benjamin twitches
When he sees me.
—*B.H.*

Allergies are the major cause of most skin rashes. An allergy is a sensitivity to a substance that causes a reaction in or on the body. Since each of us reacts differently to various substances, allergies must be treated individually. There are four kinds of allergens that cause distress:

1. Foods
2. Substances in the air (inhalants)
3. Substances that come into direct contact with the body
4. Substances that enter the body (medications, insect bites)

Food allergies are common. Chances are you know someone who can't eat strawberries without getting a rash. Or seafood. Certain foods can cause miserable itching in the rectal area

—most especially coffee, tomatoes, colas, tea, beer and choco-late. Obviously, if you suspect that your itching or your hives is caused by a certain food, eliminate it from your diet. If the symptoms persist, sit down and make a list of all the foods you've eaten within the last seven days. (A challenge to your memory!)

Show the list to your doctor. It may give him a clue to the food that is causing the trouble. He will treat the discomfort and provide protection against future attacks by a process called desensitization. He injects tiny amounts of the allergen under the skin, gradually increasing the amount until the body becomes accustomed to living with the allergen and produces its own protective antibodies.

Floating along in the air are other agents that can cause you to break out in a rash. Pollen, insecticides, dust, animal hairs, petroleum fumes, are just some of these inhalants that can make you itch and scratch. One way for the doctor to find out the cause of an allergy is to turn detective. Where have you been? Driving in the country? Picnicking in the woods? Going through an industrial area? Visiting the zoo? Once he has a few clues, he will probably make a series of skin tests. He scratches into the skin small amounts of different substances, or applies a patch test and watches for a reaction. If the skin develops a welt, he knows you are allergic to that material. He confirms his diagnosis by having you sniff or taste the material. Then he can clear up the allergy with treatment.

Probably the largest share of allergies, however, is caused by substances that come into direct contact with your skin. And the biggest villain in this group is *Rhus toxicodendron radicans*—or poison ivy. You can recognize the poison ivy plant by its shiny green leaves that grow in clusters of three from stems that are flecked with red. Its cousins, poison oak and poison sumac, also can cause unpleasant skin allergies. Poison oak resembles other oak leaves, but its leaves also grow in clusters of three. Poison sumac has long, slender leaves that grow in pairs from the stem. All three plants cause reactions in about 80 percent of those who come in contact with them. Poison ivy seems especially prevalent.

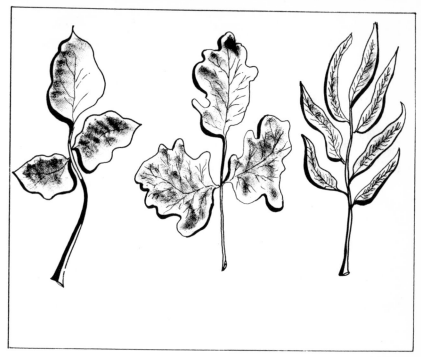

Poison ivy and its cousins, poison oak and poison sumac, are three plants that cause unpleasant skin allergies in most people. The poison ivy plant *(left)* has shiny green leaves that grow in clusters of three. Poison oak *(center)* resembles other oak leaves, but its leaves also grow in clusters of three. Poison sumac *(right)* has long, slender leaves that grow in pairs from the stem. All three plants cause reactions in about 80 percent of those who come in contact with them.

In fact, up to one million cases occur each year. Your dog may run through the underbrush and carry the poison back on his coat. Your neighbor may burn some leaves containing poison ivy that waft your way. Garden tools, clothing, shoes and gloves can carry the poison, too.

What are the symptoms? A bad case is characterized by a blistery linear rash of the skin that swells and itches like crazy. And if you succumb to temptation and scratch, your fingernails can pick up the poison and spread it to other parts of your body. An acute attack can last from two to three weeks.

Don't believe the old wives' tales about poison ivy. One attack *won't* make you immune against future ones. In fact, just the opposite is true. The first exposure to poison ivy can create a sensitivity to future attacks. And contrary to popular belief, the fluid released when a blister breaks won't start new outbreaks elsewhere. Your fingernails do the spreading. The old folk remedy of chewing ivy leaves to build up resistance to poison ivy won't work, either. It would take eight months of chewing and swallowing ivy leaves (eating more each day) to achieve a temporary immunity!

Well, what *can* you do? First and foremost, stay away from poison ivy, poison oak and poison sumac. But if you know you have been exposed, you may be able to avoid the rash if you immediately wash the exposed area with a strong household soap that has a high alkali content, then douse the area with alcohol. This treatment works only if you do it within thirty minutes after exposure to the plant. The next step, for a bad case, is to have your doctor treat your skin with soothing lotions to relieve itching. If the problem is severe, he may open bad blisters with a sterile needle and give you injections of cortisone, ACTH or antihistamines internally.

In addition to this troublesome trio, there are literally thousands of other plants and trees that can cause similar rashes in some people. If you break out in a rash after a walk in the woods, it will help the doctor in treating you if you can identify or sketch the plants and shrubs with which you came into contact.

Cosmetics are a common source of contact allergy. And since the Food and Drug Administration, at this writing, does *not* require the labeling of ingredients of nail polish, lipstick and skin products, it sometimes is difficult to pinpoint the source of an allergy. We have found that the cosmetics that most often cause contact dermatitis are nail polish, lipstick, hair dyes and bleaches, deodorants, antiperspirants, perfume, nail conditioners, depilatories, permanent waving and straightening agents, bleaching creams, face and body creams and suntanning lotions. Soaps occasionally can produce contact allergy in some people; especially those deodorant soaps containing bithionol or salicylanilide. Finally, we are now discovering allergic reactions to parabens and other preservatives used in cosmetic preparations and contact lens solutions.

Of course, the trick to successful treatment of cosmetic allergies is to detect the culprit. One young girl came into the office recently with reddened, swollen eyelids that were painfully itchy. We diagnosed the cause as her nail polish! It seems that she had the habit of scratching her eyelids with the tip of her fingernail, and the polish had caused the rash. We banned the use of nail polish for two months, used antiseptic compresses on her eyes, and applications of a cortisone ointment to clear up the rash. Then we suggested our patient use hypoallergenic nail polish. It worked just fine.

A strange case was that of the itchy skin diver. We finally traced the trouble to the medicated talcum powder he used to help him slip into his tight-fitting rubber suit!

Another young man's rash was centered on his right ear, neck and shoulder. It took several visits and many tests to determine he was allergic to his *girl friend's* hair spray. An "affectionate allergy," so to speak!

Cosmetic allergies, once they are detected and diagnosed, can be cleared up without trouble. And it is comforting to know that you can usually substitute a similar product from among the many hypoallergenic cosmetics available.

Sometimes, contact with fur, rubber, feathers, polyester, nylon or wool can cause skin rashes, too. Once diagnosed, they can be treated by your doctor. In fact, the list of possible allergies is so long it would take a whole book to discuss them. So let's move on to the last category of allergies—substances that enter the body.

Doctors know that certain drugs do cause allergic reactions in certain people, and know exactly what to do when the symptoms appear. Usually a switch from one drug or cosmetic to another of similar action will be all that's needed.

Insect bites pose a different problem. Many insects, as you know, depend upon the blood of mammals for nourishment. Some bite when they're hungry, like mosquitoes, lice and mites. Others, such as bees, hornets and wasps, attack when they're frightened. For the honeybee, that attack is fatal, incidentally. Not to you, but to the bee, since it leaves its all-important stinger behind!

Some people suffer from a fear of insects of any kind. None of us likes being bitten or stung. When an insect zeros in on you and plunges its stinger into the skin, it leaves behind a toxic substance or venom that causes the skin to swell and itch. In serious cases, there can be severe pain, even shock and unconsciousness. And you've heard of rare cases where people have had such violent allergic reactions to insect bites that they have died from the poison.

What can you do about it? Here are some sensible suggestions:

1. Know your bug. Out of the one million species of insects known to science, only a few are really out to get you. Here in the United States and Canada, the most common outdoor pests are mosquitoes, gnats, bees, wasps, yellow jackets, hornets, ticks, chiggers, fleas, ants, deer flies, bedbugs, scalp lice, itch mites and certain spider species. Of the spiders, watch out for the black widow spider, identifiable by a red, orange or yellow hourglass pattern on its belly. Its bite is *not* fatal. Another dangerous specimen is the scorpion, found only in hot, dry regions. While its sting is dangerous, producing rapid breathing and nausea, it, too, rarely produces a fatal reaction. And here's a happy thought. Most crawlers, beetles, caterpillars, praying mantises and spiders are ugly, but harmless.

2. Protect your skin. Use an insect repellent that's designed for human beings—*not* plants or household use. Available in liquid, stick, spray and impregnated tissue forms, it is easy to apply and to take with you. (And don't make the mistake that one absent-minded girl did. She thought she had packed a spray can of repellent in the picnic basket, but when the bugs began feasting on her, she took another look at the container. She'd brought her hair spray, instead.)

3. Outdoors, discourage insects by keeping food covered. Skip the perfume and aftershave, which attract bugs. Wear light-colored clothing. Don't wave your arms around to shoo away wasps and hornets. Instead, be very quiet (they are nearsighted) and put a handkerchief or scarf on a tree or bush to screen you from their view.

4. If you or a companion are stung by a bee, wasp or hornet, remove the stinger carefully. Don't squeeze it out; squeezing may cause more venom to enter the body. Ticks are tenacious and must be completely removed to avoid infection. If you can't remove the entire tick with your fingers or tweezers, touch it with lighter fluid or nail polish remover to kill it quickly (and painlessly, to you). Sizzling the tick with the flame from a cigarette lighter or match is *not* recommended, since you may get burned as well as the tick.

5. To treat any nasty bite, apply a cold compress of mild Burow's solution. If swelling appears immediately, apply ice or iced Burow's solution to the affected area.

6. If the bite itches, apply calamine lotion with phenol to the area. Slightly less effective are the old-fashioned remedies of a baking soda-and-water paste or witch hazel soothed on the area. Then, take an antihistamine.

7. If the bite is serious, a tourniquet just above the venom can prevent the poison from being absorbed into the bloodstream. Don't leave the tourniquet on too long. Take it off immediately if the skin becomes bluish and discolored.

8. If shock occurs, a doctor or ambulance should be called *at once.*

If you regularly suffer from discomfort from insect bites, visit your doctor. He can prescribe antihistamines and other medications to relieve the symptoms. In cases of severe allergy, he can desensitize your system with a series of regular injections that build up your body's immunity to the bites.

A very few people who are extremely sensitive can obtain emergency sting kits, outfitted with a syringe of epinephrine, a drug that combats severe allergic reaction.

In reading this chapter, we bet you didn't realize how many causes of itchy, reddened skin there are. Some of them, like grocer's itch, Bedouin itch and miner's itch, are caused by specialized occupations and climates, and you're not likely to encounter them! Still others are caused by worry, tension and emotional disturbances. When the cause is removed, the itches go away, too.

In certain cases, severe, prolonged itching of the skin is a danger signal that warns of internal malignancy of a body organ. If the itching lasts for several weeks, or is accompanied by bleeding, it is vital that it be diagnosed by a doctor.

A final cause of skin rashes and itches is *infection.* Infections all require a doctor's treatment and care. But to recognize the major types, here's a brief rundown of skin infections that can cause inflamed, itchy skin:

1. Eczema is a rash caused by an inherited sensitivity to certain substances. A form of allergy, it often appears in infants on the cheeks, the back of the neck and the insides of elbows and knees in the form of a red rash. Teens and adults can get eczema, too. Known medically as *atopic dermatitis,* it can be treated and kept under control with a wide variety of newly discovered medications and dieting.

2. Fungous infections can be miserable. Fungi spring to life where there's moisture, warmth, food and darkness. They thrive on the feet, the groin, under the breasts and in the armpits. And they are far more common in warm weather than in cold. Also commonly called ringworm and athlete's foot, fungous infections are stubborn enemies. However, your doctor can treat them with a combination of therapeutic measures that include compresses, fungicidal powders and ointments. There are a number of new antifungal agents that are effective against many different types of infections of the feet, hair and body. Among them are Micatin cream, Halotex and Lotrimine. Another fungicide, *griseofulvin,* is used internally; Tinactin is used externally. With these new drugs, doctors today can achieve a cure rate of about 80 percent.

3. Infectious bacteria, like fungi, require warmth and moisture to multiply. But bacteria are less sturdy and cannot stand heat. Your body usually fights bacteria all by itself with an inflammation or fever that kills off the bacteria. Sometimes, of course, the body can't cope and bacteria get the upper hand. The most common types of bacterial infections of the skin are impetigo, boils, carbuncles and *folliculitis,* which is an infection of the hair shafts, or follicles. These days, we are fortunate in being able to conquer these bacterial infections quite easily, often prescribing the use of antibiotics taken internally.

4. Venereal infections: syphilis and gonorrhea. During the past few years, owing to changing life-styles, there has been a huge rise in the number of cases of venereal disease among teen-agers. In fact, this increase is so alarming that the medical community considers these diseases to be the most severe of *all* public health problems except for upper respiratory infections.

Please learn this important fact: Use of the contraceptive Pill, which contains synthetic estrogen and progestagen, while it protects against pregnancy, does *not* give any protection whatsoever against venereal disease. Nor do any other oral or internal contraceptive devices. (For a full discussion on these pregnancy-preventers, see Chapter XVIII, *Contraceptives: What They Are, How They Work.*)

The two chief venereal diseases are gonorrhea, caused by the gonococcus bacterium, which may affect the vaginal and urethral area, and syphilis, caused by a spirochete, which usually starts as a sore on the genitals and may spread to the palms, soles and other areas of the cutaneous tissues. Fortunately, when these conditions are diagnosed early enough by a physician, and treatment is started immediately, they can easily be cured. The antibiotics most commonly used in treating them are penicillin and tetracycline. It is not advisable, under any circumstances, to resort to self-treatment, as toxic effects may occur.

We wish we could print this advice in big, red letters! If you notice any unusual sore or bodily discharge, seek professional treatment at once. If for any reason you don't have a family doctor, go to the nearest venereal clinic or hospital out-patient facility. Don't delay seeking professional help; the longer you wait, the more difficult the cure becomes.

5. Viruses, called the invisible invaders, are the tiniest enemies of the body. They are responsible for measles, mumps, chicken pox, hepatitis, smallpox and poliomyelitis.

Particularly nasty viruses are Herpes types I and II, venereal diseases that are rapidly reaching epidemic proportions. Herpes type 1 *(herpes simplex)* afflicts the face, specifically the lips, chin and cheeks. Herpes type 2 *(herpes progenitalis)* involves the genital area (the male penis, the female vagina). It is highly infectious and is transmitted through sexual intercourse. Its symptoms are itching and burning of the genital area, followed by the appearance of crops of blisters, which form a crust. The disease usually runs its course in one to two weeks. There is no effective cure or treatment for herpes, although application of ether, acetone and adrenalin may curb the duration of the disease.

Other viruses cause fever blisters, cold sores, shingles *(herpes zoster)* and even warts. Each of these can be treated by your doctor with medications and healing creams. Prevention of such viruses as smallpox and poliomyelitis can be achieved through vaccinations. Incidentally, we should mention that polio, once almost wiped out as a disease in the United States through widespread use of the Salk and Sabin vaccines, is staging an unwelcome comeback. The reason appears to be that the current generation of young parents, themselves polio immune through vaccination in childhood, have become careless about having their own youngsters vaccinated. So if you aren't sure about your own status in that regard, check with your parents and doctor to make sure you have received the necessary vaccinations. If not, get them. You also must be inoculated against certain diseases, such as smallpox, when traveling abroad.

CHAPTER FIVE
SUNTAN: DELIGHT OR DANGER?

Sun worshiping today isn't a religion—it's a worldwide avocation! And whether a suntan is acquired at the beach, on the ski slopes, on the water or under a sun lamp, it has become a symbol of sexiness in all seasons of the year.

Today, doctors believe that repeated doses of the sun are potentially harmful and aging to the skin, and may cause certain skin diseases. We'll discuss these findings in detail later on. However, apart from making the "sunstruck" feel more glamorous, a suntan does have certain benefits. In moderate doses, it can help clear up skin blemishes and acne, dry a too-oily skin, encourage the body's buildup of vitamin D and improve blood circulation. It is also good for treating *psoriasis,* a skin disease characterized by red, scaly patches.

First things first. Do you know *why* your skin changes color when you've been exposed to the sun? In the first chapter, you read that the cells of the outer layer of the skin (stratum corneum) are constantly being replaced by new, active cells that move up from the lower layers. When exposed to sunlight, the top layer of the skin thickens to screen out further burning rays.

A second process also occurs as you sit in the sun. The skin-coloring pigment, melanin, is produced in larger quantities, travels upward to the skin surface and, as a result, darkens your skin.

The production of melanin in the skin is still something of a mystery. It is known to be regulated by three hormones, and the amount of melanin in each individual skin determines whether you will tan or burn.

Sandra, for instance, is a blue-eyed blonde with a fair complexion. She naturally has less melanin in her skin and will tend to burn very rapidly when she's exposed to the sun. Her classmate Chris has brown eyes, dark hair and an olive skin. His skin produces more melanin and he will tan quite easily without going through the sunburn stage. Redheaded Pat, on the other hand, is called "Freckle Face" by her friends because sunlight causes her melanin production to concentrate in tiny clusters of suntan spots. (Freckles are simply small spots of tan caused by irregular distribution of melanin in the skin.) Robert, who is black, has the most amount of melanin in his skin. But he, too, tans, and must take precautions against overexposure just as his fair-skinned friends do.

The protective thickening of the outer layer of the skin to screen the sun's rays, combined with increased production of melanin to darken the skin, determines your own ability to tan (or burn, as the case may be). Some skins may turn toast-brown, others golden, some shocking pink. Today, however, skin specialists can gauge the sun's effect on different skin types accurately enough to advise the amount of daily exposure that will produce a tan without danger.

We've mentioned that overexposure to the sun can produce dangerous effects upon the skin. And we urge you to be aware of them. Perhaps the disease that looms largest is skin cancer. We know that constant and excessive exposure to the sun over a long period of time makes the skin more susceptible to the disease. Texans, for example, are far more likely candidates for skin cancer than Alaskans. So are outdoor people, like farmers and postmen. And while the National Cancer Institute has shown in a series of studies that one bad case of sunburn will not lead to skin

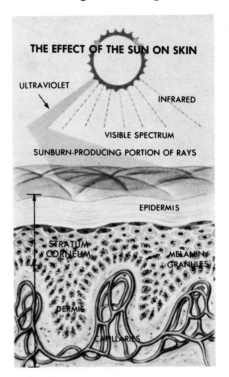

THE EFFECT OF THE SUN ON SKIN

ULTRAVIOLET

INFRARED

VISIBLE SPECTRUM

SUNBURN-PRODUCING PORTION OF RAYS

EPIDERMIS

STRATUM CORNEUM

MELANIN GRANULES

DERMIS

CAPILLARIES

(Courtesy of Today's Health, *published by the American Medical Association)*

cancer, it does warn that skin cancer can occur as a result of prolonged exposure. In other words, the more careless tanning you do, over a long period of time, the more risk you take. In fact, one expert, Dr. Joseph B. Jerome of the American Medical Association, said recently, "Sunning should be done only with proper protection for your skin, because that sun damage is cumulative . . . and there's no reversing it."

If you are freckled, with freckles that persist and grow larger as you grow older, you should be very careful about the sun, since continued irritation of these freckles by the sun's ultraviolet rays may possibly result in skin cancer.

A reassuring thought: Skin cancer is rarely fatal, and most

cancers of the skin surface can be removed surgically with complete success.

What are some of the other diseases that may occur with overexposure? *Vitiligo* is one. It is the name given to the white or "no-color" areas that may appear on the hands and face. It is the opposite of freckling and is caused by a lack of pigment cells. When the skin becomes sunburned or tanned, these surrounding spots stand out conspicuously. As a result, people with vitiligo should avoid excessive exposure to the sun and take protective measures whenever possible.

A rash, known as *polymorphous light eruption,* sometimes appears on skin that is exposed to the sun. This skin rash is produced by certain ultraviolet rays in sunlight and is aggravated by continuous reexposure to the sun. Often called an allergy to light rays, it can be prevented in some cases by taking Plaquenil tablets before going outdoors.

Chloasma, commonly known as "liver spots," may be a reaction of the skin to sun exposure. It is also seen in pregnancy. Characterized by patches of darkened skin, chloasma is caused by clusters of melanin granules and has nothing at all to do with the liver. Occurring more often among women than men, chloasma should be treated by a skin specialist.

Most of us won't have to worry about these special dangers. By following some simple precautions, we can prevent burning and achieve a suntanned skin that's healthful and attractive. How? We recommend these ten important points:

1. Consider your location. The sun is hottest closest to the equator. If you're high above sea level, the sun's rays are more powerful because there is less atmosphere to filter the sun's rays. Sunlight bouncing off water, snow or sand can cause double trouble.

2. Watch the weather. Cloudy, overcast weather still admits plenty of the sun's ultraviolet rays. Even on a completely cloudy day, 50 percent of these rays are getting through. On a hazy day, virtually all the ultraviolet light penetrates. Actually, the days when you are most susceptible to tanning are the days when there are just enough clouds in the sky to cause the sun's rays to bounce off the clouds and beam back down to earth.

3. Know what time it is. The sun's rays are strongest from noon until two in the afternoon, so either avoid sunning at that time, or cover up with protective clothing and guard your skin with a sunscreening agent.

4. Limit your tanning time. Experts all agree that on your first exposure to the sun, you should be especially careful. Extrasensitive, fair-skinned people should spend only fifteen to thirty minutes the first day, while normal and oily skin types and those with dark skins can spend up to forty minutes. On each subsequent day, increase the tanning time by fifteen minutes daily. At the end of three days the actual tanning process begins. By the fifth day, a deeper tan will become evident.

Please don't do what one young woman did. She had scrimped and saved for a glamorous two-week Caribbean cruise. With a brand-new wardrobe and high hopes, she spent her first two days on the ship's sun deck, soaking up the sun's rays. The next twelve days she spent visiting the sick bay, suffering from a serious burn and dehydration of her body fluids. Her cruise clothes stayed in the suitcase because it was torture to put them on. As she told us later, the only palm trees she saw were on postcards!

5. Protect your skin with a chemical sunscreen. As you've seen, exposure to the sun's rays is a cumulative aging process that dries the skin. (An extreme example is known as "alligator skin.") So, no matter what your natural skin color or skin type, you want to filter the sun's rays and keep your skin soft, naturally moist and pliable. There are literally hundreds of tanning preparations on the market, designed to do different tanning jobs.

In general, these formulas are based on the principle of the Angstrom, a measurement unit for wavelengths. It has been determined that rays of the ultraviolet spectrum which fall within a range of 2,900 to 3,400 Angstrom units cause tanning. Virtually all sunscreens contain PABA (para-aminobenzoic acid), derivatives of tannic acid, which comes from oak bark, as well as salt compounds called salicylates, vitamin B compounds and glycerol, which is based on glycerin.

Check the accompanying chart to determine the type that is best for your own needs.

6. Dress sensibly for sun exposure. If you're just starting a tan, take along a cover-up, wide-brimmed hat, umbrella, parasol or other means of protecting yourself against overexposure. And even if you're well tanned, you'll want some sort of protection after several hours of sun. The colors you wear matter, too. While white does reflect sunlight, darker shades do a better job of blocking ultraviolet rays. So you might want to wear a loose-fitting top in a light color, with a darker garment underneath. And remember that white clothing (especially a tee shirt) is even less protective when wet.

7. Take special care of your skin and hair. As you've seen, the sun is extremely drying. When you are hot, your body's moisture escapes in the form of perspiration. In hot sunlight, this perspiration dries so quickly on the skin surface that you often aren't aware of perspiring. Too much exposure also can coarsen your skin, leaving both hair and scalp ultradry. After sunning is the time to use the moisturizing, lubricating cleansers and lotions, dry-hair formula shampoos, conditioners and creme rinses. For many, an emollient cream applied to the skin at bedtime is especially beneficial in retaining moisture and natural oils. Mineral oil and special emulsifiers also are helpful.

8. Treat a bad sunburn medically. If you find yourself baked to a crisp after a day in the sun—and most of us do at some point—take a cool bath to wash away the skin's accumulation of grime and lotions. Then treat a mild or moderate burn with any of these measures: cool compresses of Burow's solution (one tablespoon to a quart of cool water); witch hazel or calamine lotion containing phenol; or benzocaine ointment. To dull pain, try taking a couple of aspirin or antihistamine tablets. If the sunburn persists and if the skin begins to blister, see your doctor. He can prescribe a number of medications that will ease severe pain and discomfort.

9. Use sun lamps safely. Every year, several thousand Americans must receive emergency treatment for severe sun-lamp burns and eye injuries. Experts at the Food and Drug Administration advise using sun lamps in small doses. They advocate sun lamps with automatic timers that shut off the lamp after ten minutes or less, and they advise protecting eyes with opaque plastic eye shields or dark sunglasses. If you have a skin that's sensitive to light, check with your doctor to see whether you should use a sun lamp. He can also tell you whether any medication you are taking can cause an allergic reaction to light. The FDA also reminds us that sun-lamp exposure—like exposure to the rays of the real sun—can cause premature aging of the skin and lead to possible skin cancer.

10. Be aware of heat emergencies. When the body becomes overheated, there are two real dangers. One is heat exhaustion. Its symptoms are weakness, nausea and pale, clammy skin. It is treated by getting the victim to a cool place and giving lots of fluids. A victim who still seems feverish and confused should be taken to a hospital or emergency clinic for treatment.

The other danger is heat stroke. It is the second largest cause of death among high school athletes! Last year, some 4,000 Americans, many of them teen-agers, died of heat stroke. Its symptoms are headache, weakness and confusion, with the body temperature rising sharply to 105° F. or higher. The skin becomes hot and dry. Heat stroke always should be treated in a hospital immediately. If necessary, while waiting for an ambulance, the victim should be stripped and his body submerged in a tub filled with ice cubes or ice water.

To avoid such heat emergencies, stay out of the sun from noon to two P.M., drink lots of water and liquids like Gator-ade and Sport-ade to replace body fluids and salt lost through perspiration.

To summarize, the effect of the sun on the skin can be both good and bad. Whether suntan is a danger or a delight is up to you. With sensible precautions, the sun can be a good friend that can add to your own good looks.

SUNTAN PREPARATIONS

TYPE	HOW THEY WORK	SOME TYPICAL PRODUCT NAMES
Sunscreens	Block out the sun's ultraviolet rays while permitting the skin to tan gradually; provide from maximum to medium protection, depending upon the individual formula; are safe and effective for most skin types; come in cream, lotion, gel, spray and oil form	Coppertone Shade 6 (maximum); Avon Sun Safe; Bain de Soleil; Braggi Sun Bronzing Gel, Oil, Stick; Bronze Lustre Moisturizing Tanning Gel; Bronzetan Cream Lotion; Coppertone Suntan Cream; Revlon Sun Bath Moisturizing Tanning Cream; Estée Lauder Dermatan; Sundare Clear Lotion; Sunswept, PreSun; Eclipse, Sundown

Sunblocks	Work to screen out all the sun's rays: for those who have very fair skin, blond or red hair, sensitive skin, or are freckle-prone, they provide complete protection against both burning and tanning; for those who are allergic to the sun, there are also hypoallergenic sunblocks available	Maxafil, Block Out, Solar, Solbar, SunGard, Uval
Physical barriers	Coat the skin surface, and also offer maximum protection against ultraviolet rays; are most often used by those who are outdoors in sunlight continuously, such as lifeguards and ski instructors; preparations are visible when used on the skin	RVP-Red Veterinary Petrolatum, zinc oxide ointment, A-Fil

TYPE	HOW THEY WORK	SOME TYPICAL PRODUCT NAMES
Artificial tanners ("instant tans")	Contain dihydroxyacetone, or DHA, which combines chemically with the skin's amino acids to produce a darker skin tone; since they are skin "stains," they produce only temporary coloration, and wear away as the surface skin cells do—in about four or five days; do not offer any protection against the sun's ultraviolet rays, unless they also contain a sunscreen agent, or are used in combination with a separate sunscreen product	QT-Quick Tanning Lotion, Sea & Ski Indoor/Outdoor Lotion
Lubricating and moisturizing agents	Also offer no protection against burning rays—all they do is soften the skin. Range from a number of brands of "cocoa butter" formulas to "home brews" of mineral oil, baby oil mixed with iodine, olive oil and any number of lubricating creams and lotions	Many brands, including Coppertone Cocoa Butter, Sea & Ski Tanning Butter, After Tan, Super Moist

| Internal preparations | Scientists have long been searching for a "suntan pill": one, 8-MOP, which was widely investigated some years ago, works by modifying the skin's reaction to sunlight, but extensive testing revealed unpleasant side effects; antimalarial drugs (quinine, atabrine) were also found to have powerful sunscreen properties, but they too are not recommended since they are very potent drugs and can cause liver damage, particularly in children and young people | Not recommended: 8-MOP, Atabrine, Quinine
Recommended: Trisoralen |

CHAPTER SIX
CRISP AND CLEAN

If you were confronted by a bubbling cauldron of animal fats and chunks of charred wood and ashes, would you eat it? Use it for fuel? Wash with it? Give it back to the witches?

If you had happened to be a primitive man or woman, you would have bathed with it. That ugly-smelling, mushy mess was an ancient version of soap. In matters of cleanliness, the world has come a long way.

Many early civilizations had remarkably modern methods of keeping clean. Recently, archaeologists excavated a city in Pakistan that was designed and built about 3000 B.C. On its neatly planned streets, residents dwelt in handsome homes of glazed brick. In each house were a private bath, plumbing fixtures and a waste-disposal system. Beneath the streets ran an efficient maze of culverts, pipes and water mains. In this city of Mohenjo-Daro, 5,000 years ago, children played with tub toys. Small clay figurines, made with waterspouts, were found in the bathrooms of this ancient "modern" city.

Better known to all of us are the enduring public baths of Rome, which a visitor can see there today. To the Romans, bathing was a sociable occasion which they enjoyed each day. In the large pools which held several hundred people at a time, they exchanged news and gossip as they splashed about.

When barbaric hordes from the north descended and dimmed out the light of European civilization, cleanliness became a lost secret. The splendid baths were thought of as wicked symbols of the defeated. During the Middle Ages, bathing was considered downright unhealthy. As a result, uncleanliness contributed to the terrible plagues that wiped out hundreds of thousands of people in medieval times.

Several hundred years later, in the most elegant courts of Europe, bathing was thought of as being quite eccentric—when anyone bothered to think of it at all! Beneath their gorgeous silks, satins and brocades, the blue bloods were pretty grimy. One diarist of the time, in describing the life at the French court, tells of the bejeweled ladies plastered with paints and powders that could not conceal the running sores that covered their skins. (A doctor today would diagnose the cause as accumulated dirt that bred bacteria and caused disfiguring infection of the skin.)

Even during our own Civil War, in which more American lives were lost than in any war we've fought, a tragically high percentage of the casualties was due to uncleanliness, lack of sanitation and neglect of the simplest principles of hygiene.

Today, we take cleanliness for granted. Soap, tub and shower are so much a part of our lives that we rarely give them a thought. Yet the simple ritual of washing ourselves, our clothing and the areas in which we live controls disease and wipes out germs and viruses by the millions.

Soap and water don't kill bacteria all by themselves. What they actually do is to loosen grime and dirt that accumulate on the skin. This dirt is a breeding ground for bacteria and viruses. When the dirt is rinsed away, harmful bacteria, skin-cell debris and the outer layer of skin oil are flushed away, too.

Bathing has many health benefits. Dust, smog, insecticide sprays and other skin irritants are removed when you wash. Warm water opens up the pores, dilates the blood vessels and relaxes the body tissue. Soap and water are vital to the health of your skin.

And speaking of soap, what is it? No longer the mushy mixture of primitive people, it still contains the basic elements they used. It is a mixture of alkali and fats. When boiled together, they produce glycerin and fatty acids, which combine to produce soap. You have literally hundreds of soaps from which to choose. The important thing is to choose the one that's right for you and your skin.

Among the basic types of soaps are *antiseptic* soaps that have an ingredient such as hexachlorophene to inactivate germs, *acne* soaps that contain drying agents such as sulfur and salicylic acid, and *abrasive* soaps for heavy-duty scrubbing. Often used in industrial plants, abrasive soaps may contain aluminum oxide particles, fused metal particles or oatmeal grains. *Floating* soaps, incidentally, contain no special ingredients at all. They are frothy mixtures of soap and air. The tiny air bubbles give them buoyancy. *High-sudsing* soaps contain added amounts of detergents. *Perfumed* soaps contain fragrant essences and oils that are pleasant to the nose but very often are irritating to the skin. *Superfatted* soaps have oil or lanolin added, and *hypoallergenic* soaps are cleansers that contain no irritants to cause possible allergies.

Why is one bar of soap priced at several dollars and another at a few cents? Usually, the difference lies in the amount and quality of the perfume used, advertising and packaging costs and the milling process. Expensive soaps are fine-milled, which means they retain their shape and consistency, while inexpensive soaps may become soft and shapeless in use. From a medical point of view, though, a reasonably priced white castile soap is just as good for the skin as, and sometimes better than, the most luxurious toilet soap.

A "soap" that is not a soap is a *detergent.* Detergent formulas substitute synthetics for animal fats, and these cleansers come in liquid, powder and solid forms. A liquid detergent cleanser is sometimes prescribed for acne sufferers, and usually contains hexachlorophene, petrolatum and emulsifying agents.

Cleansing creams and lotions play an important part in removing grime and makeup from the skin. These usually combine a detergent with a wetting agent. Some have lubricants added to soften the skin. Their advantage lies in the speed with which you can whisk off makeup and the fact that you can use them without water. For people with problems of too-oily or too-dry skins, the doctor may suggest a medicated cleansing cream or lotion for cleansing, along with the regular soap-and-water routine.

So much for soap and such. Let's turn to the other half of the combination: water.

What's so important about water? As we've seen, it is the rinsing agent that removes dirt, wastes and bacteria from the skin. Water is available hot, warm, lukewarm, tepid and cold. It may be hard or soft. You can use it in a bathtub, shower or basin. Millions of fighting men, in fact, have washed with the aid of a steel helmet.

How can water help your skin most? Some of the answers may surprise you. First of all, you can bathe too often. In winter, especially, too-frequent bathing can make the skin dry, flaky and itchy. In cold weather we perspire less, spend more time in dry, heated buildings and our skin supply of natural oils decreases. If your skin tends toward dryness and irritation in the winter, substitute a shower or sponge bath for the daily tub bath and save the tub for those couple of times during the week when you want to relax and take plenty of time.

A good deal of the benefit of a tub bath is psychological. In relaxing the body, it relaxes the mind. It can make you feel less tired, and lure you toward a good night's sleep. For women, it's a beauty treatment time, too. It gives gals an opportunity to scrub heels, elbows and toes, give themselves a back treatment, begin a manicure or pedicure, and even a facial! But a word of warning. *Moderate* water temperature is most healthful for the skin. If you're going to soak for a good long time, keep the temperature medium to lukewarm, especially before bedtime.

Extremes of very hot water and very cold water can cause permanent thermal damage to the skin and reduce the natural oils that keep the skin soft and supple. Instead of an icy shower, try a cool shower followed by a brisk rubdown with a towel. This combination stimulates the glands and nerves, the blood vessels contract and the body begins to manufacture oils to replace those that have been washed away.

Showers, of course, get your body cleaner more quickly than tub baths. The circulating action of the shower rinses away soap and dirt fast, while in a tub the dirt and soap stay suspended in the water all around you. The Japanese, among others, believe it unclean to combine cleansing and bathing. They soak in the tub *after* they have soaped and rinsed their bodies.

Sponge baths are less efficient than tub baths or showers because it is harder to rinse away the dirt and soap thoroughly. But they certainly are better than no bathing at all, and are useful when you're ill, or traveling in the cramped quarters of a plane or train.

Bathing regularly is an essential health habit for cleanliness. The techniques are pretty much up to the individual, though obviously it makes sense to work from the top down! And of course you pay special attention to the hidden, creased areas of the body—armpits, groin, between the toes—where accumulated perspiration and wastes should be rinsed away. During the menstrual period, doctors usually advise women to take showers rather than tub baths.

So far, we have you, the soap and the water. Anything else? According to the advertisements, there are dozens of other items to add to the bath. Three of them are essential:

1. Washcloth or bath sponge. Each has a slightly abrasive surface that removes grime and stimulates the skin surface.
2. Long-handled bath brush. The back is a breeding ground for minor blemishes, pimples and blackheads because it's so hard to reach. A bath brush keeps your back clean and smooth.
3. Thick, absorbent bath towel. After a bath or shower, always leave your skin thoroughly dried, stimulated and refreshed with a brisk toweling-off. And need we say that a towel, like a washcloth, should be your own personal property and should not be shared with others?

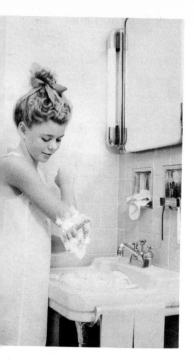

When washing, don't neglect out-of-the-way spots such as back and elbows. A long-handled bath brush is best for your back, while a hand-size brush makes quick work of elbows and knees. If hard water is a problem in your area, add a water-softening product or detergent bar to prevent skin irritation and increase lathering action of the soap. *(Cleanliness Bureau Photo)*

A tub bath, in addition to getting you clean and relaxing mind and muscles, can be a beauty treatment, too. Using a towel to cradle her head comfortably, this teen is resting her eyes with pads soaked in witch hazel. Her bath tray has a complement of aids for cleanliness and beauty, including brushes, sponge, bath oil and pumice stone. *(Cleanliness Bureau Photo)*

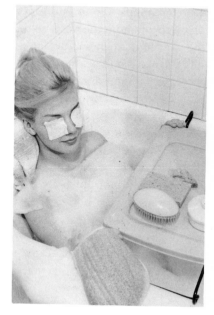

In some areas of the country, water is hard. Because it has a high alkali content, with higher amounts of calcium and magnesium, it may irritate the skin and cause soap to lather poorly. If you have this problem, add a water-softening product to your tub bath to make cleansing the skin easier and pleasanter.

In the myriad of products designed for use in the bath, some are sensible, some are fun and some are silly. Useful, for instance, is a pumice stone for rubbing away callused spots on heels and elbows. Fun are bath salts and bubble bath liquids. Inflatable backrests, headrests and trays also come under the heading of fun—if you plan to spend a lot of time in the tub! One famous musical comedy actress recently had a bath desk designed, where she catches up on her correspondence, writes out checks and even typewrites.

One bath product, however, deserves a brief paragraph to itself. Bath oils, extravagantly advertised as beautifiers and revitalizers of dry, irritated skin, are of temporary value as skin lubricants. Composed of either mineral or vegetable oils, they usually are combined with an emulsifier that distributes the oil in tiny drops throughout the water so that the oil clings to the skin. Since the skin must manufacture its own oils internally, any external oils will have only a short effectiveness. However, for dry skins they are pleasant and safe to use.

Cleanliness brings us to a problem that troubles many teens. We're talking about perspiration. Profuse perspiration and perspiration odor do cause many young people a lot of worry. Many of them have discussed it with us in the office. We explain that, first of all, perspiration is not really a problem at all. It is a normal and important body function.

Suppose your body were a balloon. If the internal temperature of your body were raised sharply by hot weather, physical activity, fever or extreme tension, your body would swell up and up and finally burst. But because the skin is naturally stretchy and because it has sweat glands that give off body heat in the form of perspiration, internal pressures don't build up to dangerous levels. So perspiration is a vital safety valve of the body.

Perspiration comes from two types of sweat glands. The larger ones are called *apocrine* glands. They are located in the armpits, the ears, the nipples of the breasts and near the sex organs. These apocrine glands are the ones that exude an odor.

Each of us also has about a million smaller glands of the *eccrine* type that produce most of our perspiration. This type of perspiration is practically odorless, and is composed of 98 percent water and 2 percent chemicals.

When you were a child, your eccrine glands did all your perspiring. Then, when you entered your teens and your body began to mature, your apocrine glands sprang into activity. For many people, the teen years are the years of heaviest perspiration flow and odor because of the physical and emotional changes that occur.

If perspiration odor troubles you, or you feel you perspire heavily, is there anything you can do about it?

Obviously, the daily bath or shower is one step. You wash away the body waste and chemical residue that collect on the skin when perspiration evaporates. Bath soaps containing hexachlorophene are good for this purpose.

Use of a deodorant chemical between baths is another step. There are three main types that can be used by a teen of either sex. It's up to you to decide which one is best for you.

1. Antiperspirants act by closing the pores and preventing the sweat glands from secreting perspiration. The ingredient that closes the pores is an aluminum salt, and it must appear on the product label as an active ingredient. Because antiperspirants do interfere with a necessary body function, they should be used only under the arms and never on any other part of the body. These aluminum salts also form acids that may irritate the skin and weaken fabric. So if you want to use an antiperspirant, follow the directions carefully and stop using it immediately if your skin becomes itchy, sore or inflamed. You'll also find it works most effectively if you apply it at night, when the skin is dry.

2. Deodorants neutralize the odor of perspiration on the body with ingredients such as hexachlorophene, neomycin, bithionol and chlorophyll. They do not close the pores, and are generally good for those who do not perspire heavily. Available in stick, spray, powder, liquid and cream form, they are the most widely used of the deodorant products by both men and women.

3. Perspiration-checking deodorants are a combination of the two types above. If they contain active aluminum salts, they should be used with care.

A third step in dealing with perspiration is to be sure that your clothing is clean and well aired after wearing. Perspiration odor can linger in a shirt, jacket or sweater unless you keep the garment as crisp and clean as you are.

And while we're on the subject of cleanliness, we'd like to mention oral hygiene. Although we're not going into detail on the importance of caring for your teeth and gums, we'd like to review the basics.

Regular dental care is a must. Every time you eat a mouthful of food, some food particles are going to roost there. These particles, when they come into contact with the bacteria in your mouth, turn into acids which begin immediately to attack the enamel on your teeth. These acids, which lodge in the pits and crevices of your teeth, start decay and gum infection if they are not removed.

You remove the acids by brushing your teeth after eating. You can't catch all of them this way, however. So you trot off to your dentist every few months for a thorough cleaning and check for cavities. You massage your gums, you brush with a good dentifrice and you stay away from the decay-building foods. Your dentist can be a good friend to you and your teeth. The dentist will show you—if you don't already know–proper brushing and massage techniques, and will recommend an effective toothpaste or powder and mouthwash.

Bad breath happens, at one time or another, to everyone. Often, it's caused by eating a spicy food or beverage or by excessive smoking. You can rid yourself of it quickly with a mouthwash rinse, a mint tablet, even a sprig of parsley. In other cases, though, bad breath may be a warning symptom of a more serious problem. If you find the trouble persisting, make a date with your dentist. It may be the sign of bad gums, decaying teeth or a mouth infection. Sometimes, infected tonsils or a queasy stomach will be the cause. In any case, you should check it out with a professional. Enough said.

Feeling scrubbed, shining and healthy? We certainly hope so! Now the next chapter is for the females in the audience. It's about the embellishments you can add to those scrubbed, shining faces—the wonderful world of cosmetics. (Gentlemen, you may join us if you wish. It *might* be very instructive!)

CHAPTER SEVEN
MOSTLY FOR MISSES

Makeup is a fascinating subject. It is an ancient art, having been practiced by both men and women since earliest times. Its evolution is traced through religious rites, tribal conflicts and the continuing wish to make the user more desirable to others.

In the twentieth century there have been decades when the style was to wear a lot of makeup. During the late 1960s and early 1970s, girls tended to the opposite extreme. As we write this, the trend is toward makeup subtly applied, to enhance natural good looks.

How important is makeup? For one thing, a good job of makeup can be significant in the job market. A recent study was made for Fairleigh Dickinson University, in which prospective employers were shown photographs of the same applicant for a secretarial job. One photograph showed her without makeup; the other, with makeup carefully applied. The result was that the employees agreed that the well-groomed, well-made-up girl would be offered 50 percent more in salary!

The goal of makeup is to emphasize your looks so that people notice *you* and not the cosmetics. The word *cosmetics* is derived from the Greek word *kosmos,* meaning adornment. We use the word today for hundreds of preparations that are rubbed,

54

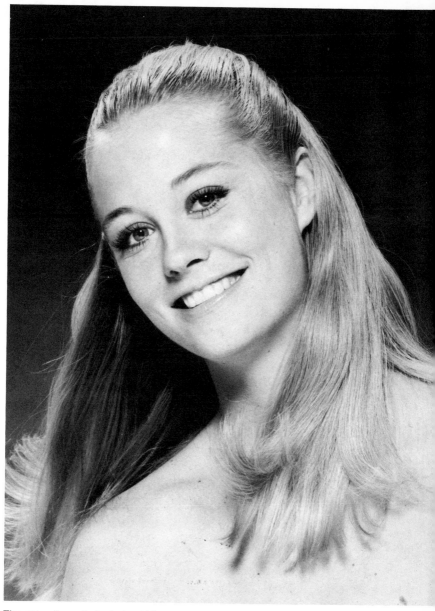

The naturally pretty look should be your goal. Use cosmetics wisely so that people notice *you*—not the cosmetics! *(Courtesy of Clairol, Inc.)*

splashed, powdered, blended and sprayed onto the skin. So let's take a closer look at cosmetics, their selection and use, and what they can do for (and to) you.

1. Foundations are actually face powders dispersed in an alcoholic, watery, glycerin base. When applied to the skin, foundations dry almost immediately. In liquid and cream formulas, they are used under powder to cover the skin and produce a smooth matte finish. For young skins, foundations should not be necessary during the daylight hours. For evening wear and special occasions, they can add an extra bit of glamour.

2. Pressed powders are what they sound like—loose powder (talcum, starch and stearates) pressed into solid cake form. Many pressed powders are a mixture of powder plus foundation, combining the coverage of a base and the clinging power of powder. These are suitable for everyday use and are easy to apply. Never use a powder-plus-foundation over regular foundation. The result would be heavy and "masky" looking.

3. Loose powders, like pressed powders, are composed of talcum, starch and stearates. They give the skin a fine texture, absorb oils and keep makeup looking fresh. Available in many shades, they can give the skin a translucent look that is especially attractive at night. Loose powder should be used over a foundation, cream or skin lotion for staying power. And you should always powder generously, whisking off the excess with a cotton square or complexion brush for a perfectly smooth finish.

4. Foundation sticks come in stick form or in lipstick-type tubes. They are *concentrated* foundation lotions with sulfur and hexachlorophene added to them. Use them to cover up and help heal minor skin blemishes, or, in unmedicated form, to disguise dark shadows under the eyes.

5. Blushers and glossers color and tint the skin temporarily. Used sparingly, they highlight eyes and facial contours and give a pleasing glow to the face. In many shades, ranging from the beige browns through coral, pink and red, they can be used over the foundation and under the powder or as a finishing touch over makeup. For evenings or on "pale days" when you look washed out, a bit of color is very flattering, as long as it looks like *you*.

6. Astringents are liquids applied on your "bare" face, before you apply makeup. They brace the skin, temporarily close the pores and remove excess surface oils or sebaceous secretions. Composed of alcohol, water, aluminum, perfume and antiseptic, they are especially useful for oily skins. A natural astringent, which can be used for the same purpose, is witch hazel.

7. Hand and body lotions are used to combat dryness, chapping and skin irritation. They usually contain mineral or vegetable oil, cetyl alcohol, emulsifying agents, lecithin, lanolin, cholesterol, perfume and distilled water. In some formulas, vitamins A, D and E are added, along with pantothenic acid derivatives, for added skin benefits. For those with normal or dry skin, these lotions also are good makeup bases under regular powder or pressed powder, since they are nondrying.

8. Cold creams are a fluffy mixture of beeswax, oil, borax, alcohol and water. They often are called all-purpose creams because they temporarily soften the skin, remove makeup and smooth the skin surface. Variations of cold cream are called night creams or emollient creams. (Cold cream, by the way, is a highly effective remover of eye makeup.)

9. Cleansing lotions or creams usually are a combination of a detergent and a wetting agent. They are useful when traveling, or when you want to remove makeup in a hurry without water. (You can achieve the same results, though, with mild soap, water and a bit more patience.)

10. Lipsticks come in literally hundreds of shades, in the familiar stick, liquid and pencil forms. Made from beeswax and lanolin, their colors come from various eosin dyes. Sometimes, these dyes may produce an allergic effect and cause swelling and blistering. If this happens to you, change the color and/or brand immediately. Lipsticks come in various formulas. The so-called "permanent" lipsticks retain their color longer on the lips, but tend to be drying. Others—like lip glossers—add more oil for shine, but require frequent touch-ups. Lipstick pencils are an excellent

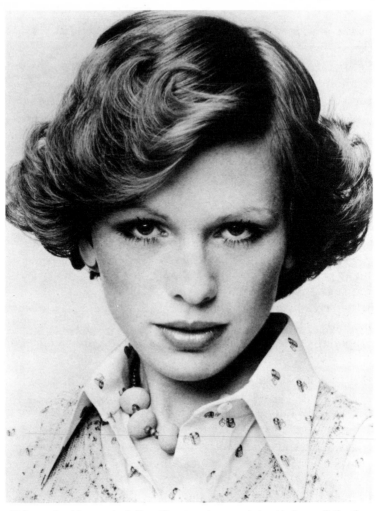

Makeup should never look "hard" or overdone, and should always fit the time and place. For daytime, a powder-plus-foundation is sparingly applied to the skin. Brows are brushed smooth with a child's toothbrush. Eyes are highlighted with a touch of mascara on upper and lower lashes. Lips are tinted with a soft shade accented by a bit of glosser. For evening, you might accent cheekbones with blusher, add a soft touch of eye shadow and apply a brighter shade of lip coloring. *(Courtesy of Clairol, Inc.)*

means of defining and shaping the lip line neatly. Use a shade darker than your lipstick, then fill in the outline with your regular lipstick or glosser.

11. Mascara is a cream containing dye that colors the ends of eyelashes and makes them look longer and thicker. (The ends of eyelashes are often sun-bleached and so aren't seen against the cheek.) Mascara comes in cream, liquid or cake form, and in a rainbow of colors. We don't think mascara is necessary for day-time unless you happen to have unusually pale or sparse lashes. For evening, mascara can look very attractive if you harmonize it with your eyes and hair coloring and don't slather it on like war paint.

12. Eyeliners also are dyes, dispersed in cream or liquid bases. In pencil form, eyeliners give the softest line and are more appropriate for daytime wear. Available in many colors, they should be used with a light touch.

13. Eye shadow is a dye suspended in a cream. It also comes in liquid and dry form. If you are using it for evening, use the cream type over your foundation before powdering. The other forms are applied over face powder. Eye shadow can enhance the eyes, but the prettiest effects are the most subtle. Soft shades, such as smoky gray, pale blue and soft turquoise, are also the most flattering to young eyes.

14. Perfumes, colognes, toilet waters and aftershaves are mixtures of essential oils, alcohol and fixatives. Perfumes contain a higher percentage of essence to alcohol, and are meant to be applied to small areas of the skin. Cologne, toilet water and aftershave contain more alcohol and are designed to be splashed liberally on the skin. Allergic reactions to some perfume products are quite common, with two essential oils, oil of bergamot and furocoumarin, often the culprits. If you have an allergic reaction to a particular brand of perfume but love its scent, try switching to the same scent in the less-concentrated cologne or toilet water form. Many find that scent in cream concentrate form is kindest to their skins.

ALLERGEN	COSMETIC PREPARATION
Aluminum salts	Deodorants, antiperspirants, astringents
Ammoniated mercury	Freckle creams, antiseptic ointments
Barium salts	Depilatories
Beta-napthol	Freckle creams
Boric acid	Lipstick formulas, baby creams
Cresylic compounds	Antiseptic household preparations
Essential oils	Perfumes, colognes, toilet waters, aftershaves, masking and deodorant agents
Formaldehyde	Antiseptic solutions, disinfectants, household deodorizers, preservatives, plastics, nail hardeners
Lanolin	Hand lotions, hair lotions, face creams
Lauryl alcohol sulfates	Shampoos, water-dispersible ointment bases
Mercuric bichloride	Antiseptic lotions, freckle creams
Phenolformaldehyde resins	Plastics
Phythalates	Insect repellents
Phenylenediamine compounds	Hair dyes, eyelash and eyebrow cosmetics
Polyethylene glycols	Pharmaceutical water-dispersible bases, cosmetic bases, wetting agents, hand lotions

ALLERGEN	COSMETIC PREPARATION
Salicylic acid	Face-peeling preparations, corn cures
Sulfur	Acne preparations, hair pomades and dressings
Thioglycolate	Permanent hair-waving lotions, depilatories
Zinc salts	Deodorants, astringents

Those fourteen different items of makeup are considered basics today. We don't suggest you need all of them. But we think it is important for you to know something about each of them so that you can make your own choices wisely and well. When you stop to think about it, cosmetics today are a far cry from the bit of rice powder and dab of rouge that your great-grandmother may have used!

Other factors determine the amount and type of makeup you should wear. Is your skin oily? Or does it tend to be dry? Obviously, oily skin types should shy away from cosmetic preparations that contain extra oils. Alcohol-based lotions and astringents are good cleansers for oily skins. Cream-type foundations and heavy makeups are not flattering to (or good for) oily skins, so avoid them. Dry skin types will find that creamy lotions and foundations help soften and smooth the skin. (For special skin routines, you might want to go back and review Chapter III.)

Girls with sensitive skins should consider the use of *hypoallergenic* cosmetics. These special cosmetics are designed for those who experience allergic reactions to other cosmetics, with formulas designed to contain the least possible amount of allergens. Manufactured by several reliable firms, these hypoallergenic cosmetics encompass the whole range of makeup items—from nail polish to lipstick.

"Natural cosmetics," derived from fruits, vegetables and

herbs, are very popular, but those with delicate and sensitive skins may suffer reaction to some of the ingredients they contain. Some beauty experts suggest do-it-yourself cleansing masques, such as puréeing a peach in the blender, applying it to the face, letting it dry, then rinsing it off. Another "natural" facial is a mixture of instant oatmeal-and-water paste which is allowed to dry on the skin, then removed with a *dry* washcloth to rid the skin surface of dry, flaky cells. A good "natural" cleanser is one cup of apple cider vinegar combined with one cup of warm water, splashed on the skin. Another treatment, said to be good for oily skins, is applying plain, chilled yogurt to the face. It contains lactic acid, which has a drying effect on surface skin oils.

Many people are allergic to some of the elements found in cosmetics. You probably know some girls who can't use a certain brand of lipstick or antiperspirant. Perhaps you've had some trouble yourself. We've compiled a list of the most common allergens and the cosmetics in which they are found. If you find that any of them are irritating to you, stop using the item! You will be able to find a similar one that you *can* use.

We advocate substituting hypoallergenic cosmetics for any cosmetic which may cause an allergic dermatitis.

Birthmarks, scars and burns can disfigure a complexion and cause a great deal of anxiety. Some skin disfigurations can be treated by a dermatologist by planing, freezing and other surgical techniques. But many can be concealed effectively with cosmetic cover-ups. One of the most famous is CoverMark, a facial cream tinted to blend with skin tones. It does an excellent job of covering even conspicuous birthmark patches. For less serious blemishes, there are many lipstick-shaped cover-up sticks, which are concentrated foundations in cream bases.

Before you begin with makeup experimentation, hold on! Always consider cosmetics in relation to your skin coloring, hair and eyes as well as your skin type. Just because Sylvia bought a beautiful pale coral lipstick that looks great on her, that's no reason to assume it will look as well on you. Nature mixed a special palette of colors and tones that add up to *you,* and no one else has coloring quite like yours. So it stands to reason that you should use colors that complement your skin. The simple table on page 64 will help you in choosing becoming shades of makeup.

In addition to your skin type and your coloring, also consider your height and build in relation to your makeup. Petite girls should scale cosmetics to their size. (Dainty, delicate features will look clownish if overemphasized.) Taller girls with bigger bone structure often can use more vivid cosmetics, boldly applied. And finally, of course, consider you and the life you lead. *Whatever cosmetics you use should fit the time and the place.* (That's a good motto to remember, always.)

Before we complete our discussion of cosmetics, let's cover a few special tips that you might find helpful. Most of you are so clever at applying makeup that we think it's superfluous to detail each step. But do you know these pointers?

1. Makeup *darkens* on the skin the longer it stays there. The combination of natural skin oils and cosmetics turns powders and foundations gradually deeper as the hours go by. So keep this factor in mind when choosing your original shade of makeup.

2. You can test a powder shade by rubbing it on the inside of the arm with a cotton pad. If the powder is too light in shade and texture, it will disappear completely into the skin. If it is too dark, too heavy or the wrong shade, it will show up startlingly on the skin. The "right" shade is the one that blends into the skin with a flattering, soft finish.

3. To cover up dark circles under the eyes, dot on a foundation that's lighter than your skin tone. Then blend it in with a cotton swab. Or use a cover-up stick or cover-up cream.

4. Even if you are "antilipstick," or have naturally rosy lips, you should always apply some sort of protection to your lips—such as glosser or Vaseline. To lighten the shade of lipstick, apply glosser first, lipstick last.

5. If you wear eyeglasses all the time, soften the look of the eye behind the lenses with eyeshadow in soft shades, extending the shadow to the brow line. Eyeliner along upper lash line adds

SKIN TONE	POWDER AND FOUNDATION	EYES	EYE SHADOW AND EYELINER	LIPSTICK AND/OR GLOSSER
Ivory	Natural, ivory, or light beige	Blue	Gray, blue, violet	Pink, blue-red, coral
Golden	Beige, rose-beige	Brown	Gray, brown, turquoise	Coral, orange, clear red
Medium	Light rachel or rose-beige	Hazel	Gray, green, brown	Pink, orange, clear red, blue-red
Ruddy	Rachel, light brunette	Blue	Gray, slate blue, violet	Blue-red, clear red
Brunette	Dark rachel, deep beige	Brown	Green, brown, turquoise	Clear red, deep orange, copper red
Olive	Dark rose-beige or brunette	Brown	Green, brown, turquoise	Coral, orange, clear red
Black	Warm brown, bronze	Brown	Brown, plum, dark green, dark gray	Russet, wine, copper red, clear red

(Keep in mind that when you have a suntan, you should choose a darker shade of powder or foundation in your same tone range to complement the change in your skin color.)

emphasis, too. For evening, apply a bit of mascara. Always make sure, in selecting eyeglass frames, that the frames and your eyebrows are in proper proportion. And to balance your face, use a bright, light shade of lipstick that emphasizes your lips.

6. For those of you who wear contact lenses, there are special precautions you must take! Be very careful about exposing the lenses to cosmetics, lotions, soaps, creams and hair sprays. Apply cosmetics only *after* inserting the lenses, and use cosmetics very sparingly around the eyelids. If you do want to use mascara occasionally, use *waterproof* mascara. Never use the "lash-extender" mascara because it contains tiny fibers that may enter the eyes and become trapped under the contact lenses. If contact lenses become filmed and clouded by cosmetics, they should be cleaned with a commercial contact-lens cleansing solution. If irritation develops, see your eye doctor immediately.

7. Makeup should never look "hard" or overdone. Learn to use cosmetic brushes for application and for blending. Cotton pads and cotton swabs also are very useful aids for applying cosmetic and eye makeup. A child's toothbrush, by the way, makes a splendid eyebrow brush.

8. Keep your makeup tools and accessories scrupulously clean. Don't share them with anyone else! A dirty powder puff, for instance, can spread dirt and oils over your skin every time you use it. Washable foam rubber puffs or cotton balls are effective substitutes. Combs, brushes and other implements you use on your face and hair should be washed regularly, too.

Makeup, as we said some pages ago, is a wonderful world to explore. But keep in mind what one young man said to his fiancée after she had spent the entire day at the beauty parlor. He took a long look at her and said: "Mmmm, you look great! Did you take a nap this afternoon?" After she got over her astonishment, she realized that he'd paid her a priceless compliment. She looked relaxed, pretty and natural.

And *that's* what makeup should do!

CHAPTER EIGHT
TWENTY TO A
TEEN– FINGERS AND TOES

Flashing on a typewriter, flying on piano keys, flipping a throw to first base, our fingers guide, grasp, stir and fling—performing many tasks that we take for granted. We also disregard our toes. Yet we've got twenty digits in all, and their care is important to health and good looks.

Our hands and fingers are busy parts of the body. Their epidermal covering (skin!) comes into contact with many objects as well as extremes of heat and cold. So it follows that they are subject to injury and special problems. Let's take a look at some typical cases in our office files.

WALLY'S WARTS

Wally had several warts on his hands, which didn't cause him any pain. But he found them annoying, ugly to look at, and wanted to get rid of them. He told us, with a big grin, that his grandmother had suggested he rub them with a raw potato. It hadn't done any good, said Wally. He also had tried using castor oil on them, which didn't work either. So he came to us.

We told him that warts are caused by a specific wart virus which causes regrowth of tissue. We explained that warts can spread by contact or rubbing with the fingers. Obviously, you can harvest quite a crop of warts by picking at them or irritating them.

Weirdly enough, the nerves and emotions seem to be tangled up with warts, too. There are many actual cases on record where warts have disappeared because of the power of suggestion of some folk remedy, such as the application of a raw potato on them. In fact, the power of suggestion can be so strong that such a renowned specialist as Dr. Bruno Bloch of Vienna has recommended hypnosis in removal of warts!

Wally's warts would probably disappear if just left alone. A good many do. But in a bothersome spot, between the fingers, for instance, where it might interfere with writing or drawing—or if it is disfiguring—a wart should be removed. Years ago a common home treatment for warts was to burn them away with nitric or sulfuric acid. This treatment often left a nasty permanent scar that looked worse than the wart. For Wally's warts, we treated them carefully with a potent chemical, trichloracetic acid. They disappeared. If warts bother you, see your doctor—he's much better able to deal with them effectively than you are.

RHODA'S RED HANDS

Rhoda, when she came into the office, was miserable. Her hands were red, swollen and painfully itchy. We did a patch test to determine whether the condition was due to a contact allergy. The test proved that she was allergic to a hair-set solution that she used every night to put up her hair. As in many cases, her scalp was not allergic to the lotion, only her hands.

Rhoda's case, luckily, was simple. But many people are allergic to other common substances such as detergents, lotions, cosmetics and household soaps, to name just a few. Even if you are not allergic, it's wise to avoid prolonged exposure to harsh cleansers and water, to avoid extremes of heat and cold and to keep hands dry to prevent chapping. Protective silicone ointments, hand lotions and creams can help prevent redness and roughness, since they help the hands maintain their own natural oil balance. The wearing of cotton-lined rubber gloves is a good idea if your hands are in water frequently. And cotton work gloves are smart for those of you who do a lot of tinkering with cars and have heavy outdoor chores.

BARNEY'S BLISTERS

"It's just a plain old blister," said Barney plaintively, as he entered the office. "But I'm on the school tennis team," he continued, "and I can't grip my racquet properly."

We examined the blister and saw that it was inflamed and irritated. So we decided to puncture it before it burst from friction and caused infection. We washed the area with soap and water and sterilized it with alcohol, then we punctured it with a sterilized needle at the side to remove the fluid that had collected under the outer layer of skin. We left the outer skin layer in place as a protective cover. And Barney soon was back in action, starring for his school.

The blister is caused by pressure and friction on a localized area of the skin. It also can be caused by a severe burn. Fluid builds up between the skin layers and continued pressure can cause a painful foot or finger. The best approach to blisters is prevention. Foot blisters can be guarded against by wearing properly fitted shoes that have enough room beyond the big toe and do not slip and chafe at the heel. Two pairs of socks for sports —sweat socks worn over a lightweight cotton pair—also help. Hands can be protected against blistering by taping with hypoallergenic adhesive or by wearing special sports gloves of the type worn by golfers. And always remember that any bad blister may become infected and so require prompt medical attention.

SALLY'S SPLIT NAILS

Sally's fingernails were soft and brittle. Several of them had split quite badly. Two had flaked, and one had broken off. This condition is not unique, we explained, and is due to a variety of causes.

Some people are born with soft nails, and there is little that can be done about it. Others have brittle nails caused by a deficient diet. Some specialists believe that split, broken nails also are a symptom of internal and external diseases. In serious cases, a doctor can identify the source of the trouble through clinical and laboratory examination.

In Sally's case, we decided her diet was at fault. Pizzas, French fries and soda pop—her favorite foods—are not high in vitamin content or balanced protein. We suggested a change in her eating habits to encourage a more balanced, healthful diet and prescribed the use of an envelope of unflavored gelatin, dissolved in fruit or vegetable juice, as a beauty appetizer to be drunk each day. We told her to keep up the regime until her next appointment three months later. And since Sally had no history of cosmetic allergy, we also suggested she use a nail polish with a special hardening ingredient to allow the nails to grow out without breaking or splitting. (Be careful about using nail-hardening polishes, especially if you have any tendency to cosmetic allergy. They can often contribute to cosmetic dermatitis.)

Nails, by the way, are quite similar to human hair, although you wouldn't guess so. Both begin deep inside the skin, both can be cut and trimmed and both depend upon the body processes for nourishment and growth. In fact, the chemical components of the nails are similar to those of the hair! Nails grow about one-quarter inch each month. They should be neatly trimmed and cared for to prevent hangnails, ingrown toenails and other annoying problems. (We'll chart out manicure and pedicure routines for both sexes at the end of this chapter.)

But now let's turn to the feet. Since our feet are used actively in walking, dancing and sports, they are prone to many disorders of the skin.

ANDY'S ATHLETE'S FOOT

Probably the most frequent infections of the skin of the feet are those caused by fungi. You remember that in Chapter IV we said that fungous organisms needed warmth, darkness and moisture in which to grow and multiply. The foot is one of the favorite breeding grounds of fungi, and so we have the ailments known as athlete's foot and ringworm, which also mean fungal and bacterial infection.

Andy's case is a good illustration of the problem. His toes were red, itchy and had blisters between them. The soles of his feet also were affected with painful, calloused lesions.

"Glad you came to see us," we told him. "If not treated, your athlete's foot becomes much harder to clear up and a related condition known as an *id dermatitis* may appear in other areas of the body, especially your hands."

The problem in treating fungous infections of the feet, as we explained to Andy, is the fact that we are dealing with a very durable organism. Attempts to destroy the organism on the skin also will destroy the skin itself. So we have to attack the fungi mildly and make the foot less inviting to the fungi as a place to breed. We prescribed this step-by-step treatment for Andy:

1. Wash the feet thoroughly, using warm water and a mild soap or detergent. Pay special attention to cleansing the area between the toes.
2. After washing, soak the feet in a medicated solution. For Andy, we prescribed Burow's solution. In other cases, we might prescribe boric acid compresses, depending upon the organisms present.
3. Dry the feet thoroughly, keeping in mind that excess moisture helps fungi to grow.
4. Place small cotton balls or squares of gauze between the toes to keep them separated and aerated.
5. Use an antiseptic powder or lotion before putting on clean socks or stockings. We gave Andy a prescription for a fungicidal ointment for this purpose. (Nonprescription medications available include antiseptic foot powders, solutions, ointments and sprays.)
6. Change shoes and socks or stockings frequently, using antiseptic powder or ointment at each change and at whatever times during the day the feet feel hot or moist. Make sure your shoes fit well and that the leather is not too stiff or heavy.

As we told Andy, if athlete's foot happens to be a problem, you have to learn to pamper your feet! You have to learn new habits of washing, drying and medicating the feet. Infected shoes should be disinfected and stockings thoroughly washed in boiling water. Shoes must be correctly fitted to the feet and their use rotated. (Switch shoe styles several times each week, for instance.) The new oral fungicide griseofulvin has been successful in the treatment of very severe cases of athlete's foot.

Bacterial infections also occur when feet suffer abrasions and cuts. If you like to pad around the house or garden in your bare feet, you may find yourself with a case of pyoderma or impetigo. They are caused when the bacteria that lie on the skin enter the bloodstream through a cut or scrape and localized or body infection occurs. These infections can be cleared up by the use of external antibiotics like neomycin and bacitracin. Internal antibiotics also can be prescribed.

You'll want to follow proper foot hygiene as we've just outlined in our discussion of athlete's foot to clear up these other infections. Also treat them by cutting down on sweets and carbohydrates in your diet, using a laxative or laxative foods to clean out the digestive tract when necessary, increasing your consumption of water and other fluids, getting plenty of sunlight, air and exercise and keeping the skin clean and dry.

IRA'S INGROWN TOENAILS

Less serious, but very painful, are ingrown toenails. Ira hobbled into the office one afternoon with an ingrown nail on his big toe. The side of the nail had begun to penetrate into the skin, making it feel sore and uncomfortable. Since the nail had not penetrated deeply into the flesh, and had not caused severe infection, we altered the growth pattern of the nail by putting a bit of medicated cotton between it and the skin. We applied antibiotic ointment and a compress to prevent reinfection. And we told Ira to keep the cotton in place until the nail grew out of the groove and had extended well beyond the toe's edge. In serious cases, when infection has set in, surgical treatment is required and sometimes it becomes necessary to cut away parts of the nail and the adjoining skin. After any surgical procedure of this kind, it's best to wear shoes that are wider in the toes to avoid too much pressure on the area. Ingrown nails are due usually to improper cutting of the toenails and tight-fitting or too-pointed shoes that don't conform to the shape of the foot.

PLANTAR WARTS

Plantar warts are an increasingly common foot problem, because young people like to go barefoot. Basically, they are no different from other warts. But their location of the sole of the foot (the plantar surface) makes walking painful because of pressure of body weight upon the foot. In some cases, they disappear spontaneously. In other cases, the pressure can be relieved by cushioning the area with a callus pad.

A plantar wart can be treated medically in several ways. The doctor may apply a bichloroacetic or trichloroacetic acid. Occasionally, weekly application of 40 percent salicylic acid plaster, left on for three days, is helpful. Usually, however, a plantar wart is removed by *electrodesiccation*. This is a process whereby the doctor injects novocaine into the area, applies an electrical current through a needle, and then scrapes the wart away.

CORNS AND CALLUSES

Corns and calluses are unpleasant foot problems that can afflict any of us from time to time. They are the skin's way of reacting to pressure because of too-tight or poorly fitted shoes. The thickness of the skin builds up both on the outer layer and inside the skin until it resembles a horny lump. You can treat calluses and corns by soaking the affected foot in hot water, applying salicylic acid to the corn or callus (sold under various trade names as liquid corn and callus removers) and surrounding the area with a protective pad for a few days to keep pressure from it. Repeated applications of hot water and salicylic acid help to soften the corn or callus until the skin turns white and dead-looking. Then this affected skin can be removed with the fingers and a terry towel, abraded with a file or cut away with a sharp knife or scalpel. If this treatment does not work, then consult a chiropodist. (And need we say that the best treatment of corns and calluses is removing the cause? Make sure that your shoes fit properly and without discomfort.)

PERSPIRATION OF THE FEET

A final foot problem is perspiration. It is a problem that is compounded by jogging, tennis and other exercise that stimulates the heavy flow of perspiration. Heavy sports socks that aren't porous and don't permit normal evaporation add to the discomfort. Poorly fitted shoes, sneakers, running shoes and boots also cause feet to perspire and create unpleasant odor.

An imbalance of the sympathetic nervous system, called *hyperhidrosis,* is a severe form of foot perspiration. Its symptoms are excessive perspiration, caused by the growth of bacterial organisms on the skin combined with the breakdown of sweat, and an accompanying offensive smell. It can be treated by washing the feet several times during the day, followed up with application of an antiperspirant and antibacterial foot powder.

So many foot disorders are related to wearing improperly fitted footwear, and to carelessness about cleanliness and grooming, that we think it's important to emphasize that *prevention* is the easiest way to foot health. Weekly home pedicures and manicures are essential, too. Here is an easy routine to follow:

NAIL GROOMING FOR MEN

Equipment

> Emery board (preferable to metal files that leave small, dirt-collecting crevices)
> Warm, soapy water and towel
> Orangewood stick for removing dirt under the nails (again, this is kinder to nails than a metal file)
> Cuticle softener
> Nail clipper

Use

Trim nails with nail clipper, then file the nails with an emery board, making sure edges and tips of nails are smooth and even. File fingernails across to a slightly rounded shape; file toenails straight across to discourage ingrown toenails. Soak fingertips and/or toes in soapy water to loosen dirt, then remove accumulated dirt under the nails with an orangewood stick. Apply a cuticle-softening lotion as directed on the label. Push back cuticle gently. Trim away excess cuticle with clippers and carefully wipe away any remaining softener. Repeat entire procedure once a week. Clean and file nails whenever needed.

NAIL GROOMING FOR WOMEN

Equipment

> Nail clipper and manicure scissors
> Emery board
> Orangewood stick
> Warm, soapy water and towel
> Cuticle softener
> Polish remover
> Nail polish in your choice of shade
> Polish base and sealer
> Cotton-tipped swabs or loose cotton

Use

Begin by removing old nail polish with remover and cotton swab or loose cotton. Then shape the tips. Trim nail ends with clipper, and file with an emery board to an oval shape. Clean under the nails with an orangewood stick. Soak fingers (or toes) for ten minutes in warm, soapy water and dry carefully. Apply cuticle softener with cotton-tipped swab or cotton-covered orangewood stick. Lavishly coat cuticle, nail and under the nail tip. Loosen cuticle around edges of the nail with orangewood stick and clip away any hangnails or loose bits of skin. Rinse and dry again. If you are going to apply nail polish (which, by the way, is a good protector against breaking and tearing), begin with a

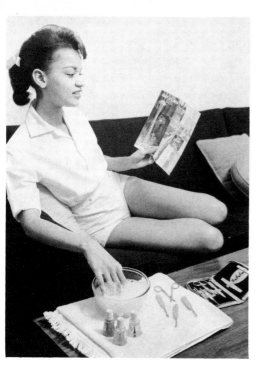

An important first step in a weekly manicure is to soak fingertips in warm soapsuds to cleanse skin and nails and to soften cuticles. Then you're ready for cuticle softener and polish. If you use polish, begin with a polish base for longer protection and good looks. *(Cleanliness Bureau Photo)*

A weekly pedicure is a must for healthy feet. Soak toes in warm, soapy water for ten minutes and smooth calluses and rough spots with a pumice stone. Dry carefully, then clean and shape nails before applying polish. To prevent the possibility of ingrown toenails, always file or clip nails straight across. *(Cleanliness Bureau Photo)*

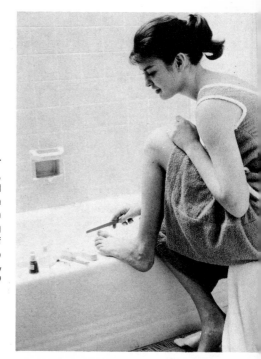

polish base. Let it dry thoroughly, then apply two coats of nail polish, painting from base to tip. Naturally, you'll allow plenty of drying time between coats. And always leave a hairline edge of natural nail showing at the tip to discourage peeling. Do this by rubbing your opposite thumb along the edge. Let polish dry completely, then apply the sealer. If you reapply a thin coat of sealer every few days, your polish job should last for a week.

FOUR TRICKS FOR HAPPY FEET

Finally, here are four simple ways to make your feet more limber, supple and comfortable. (Remember, your feet support your body weight and make good posture possible.)

1. Minute massage. After you have completed your pedicure, hold your right foot in one hand and twist the ankle to each side five times. Then, take your thumb and press it in firmly over the entire sole of the foot, starting with the toes and working back to the heel. Complete the massage by pulling each toe apart gently from the one next to it. Repeat with the left foot.

2. Toe curls. At home, sit in a straight chair with feet flat on the floor. Curl your toes under and push toward the floor until the arches lift off the floor. At the beach, curl your toes when walking in the sand, dig deep holes in the sand, pick up shells with your toes. All of these toe exercises add foot flexibility and strength.

3. Kitchen caper. Face the kitchen sink or countertop, holding on with both hands. Place your weight on your right foot. Lift your left foot and place it behind your right ankle. With the left foot pressed against the right ankle, raise yourself up and down on the toes of the right foot ten times. Shift your weight to the left foot and repeat the exercise. This strengthens ankles and arches.

4. Phonebook push-up. Stand on a telephone book with the balls of your feet resting on the phone book, heels up in the air. Lower heels to the floor as slowly as you can. Repeat several times. This exercise limbers up arches and backs of the calves.

CHAPTER NINE
WHAT'S ON TOP?

Let's, as they say in show business, start at the top. We're talking about your hair. It's a fascinating subject.

First of all, hair is a form of skin. It grows out of the body, it gets its nourishment from the body, its condition reflects the condition of the body. Amino acids and chemicals are converted into *keratin,* which forms the basis for all types of outer tissue: hair, skin, fingernails—even horns and feathers in animals.

Each hair on your body grows in an opening known as a *follicle.* From another tiny opening, the *sebaceous gland* supplies oil to the hair and skin. Together, these two openings are linked in the hair apparatus. At the bottom of the hair shaft is the *papilla,* a tiny cradle which is the manufacturing plant for the hair. The base of each hair widens to form a bulb that fits into the light socket of the papilla.

What happens if you yank out a strand of hair? Nothing. The little papilla will go right on generating and sending up a new hair to the skin surface. So there is nothing scientifically true to the phrase "pulling out a hair by its root." A healthy hair sits in its follicle, perched on the papilla, and is well nourished through the capillaries and blood vessels fed by the bloodstream. When the bloodstream provides the hair with plenty of proteins, fats, carbohydrates, enzymes and minerals, hair flourishes. If the blood is undernourished, then the hair becomes undernourished, too.

In fact, your hair reflects your body's health. Doctors use the condition of hair as a clue in determining general health and well-being. Mental tension and emotional disturbance are linked with hair health. Overactive sebaceous glands, for instance, are considered a contributing cause of common baldness. Another kind of sudden tension actually causes your hair to stand on end, as we mentioned earlier. These examples illustrate how the behavior of hair is linked with the entire nervous system.

If you were to look at one strand of hair under an electronic microscope, what would you see? You'd see something that looked a great deal like the Golden Gate Bridge! The molecules of each of the three layers of one strand of hair are linked together like a cable. Scientists believe that the hair "cable" is kept from unraveling by a continuous supply of protein. And when too much tinkering with proteins occurs, hair problems result. By tinkering, we mean the excessive use of too many hair dressings containing alcohol, solvents or oils that destroy the proteins and cause the hair "cable" to unwind.

Other factors cause hair problems, too, and we'll discuss these problems and their treatment in the following chapters.

Now let's find out how hair grows. You have from 90,000 to 140,000 hairs on your head. Each hair grows about a half-inch each month and lives from two to six years before it falls out. Those are average figures for young adults. But the rate of hair growth differs on various parts of the body, among different races, between males and females and according to age.

The hair on your head takes the longest to grow from the papilla to the surface of the scalp. Studies have shown that if a hair is plucked off the crown of your head, it will take more than four months for another hair to replace it on the skin surface, while an eyebrow hair will pop to the surface in half that time. But once the hair becomes visible, then it grows fastest on the scalp and on a man's chin. On men, underarm hair and thigh hair grow twice as fast as on women. But a feminine hair lasts about 25 percent longer than a male's. On women, hair grows fastest between the ages of fifteen and twenty-five. Its most rapid growth occurs in the summer. And believe it or not, everybody's hair grows a bit faster at night!

The color of your hair is determined by chemical oxidation and dispersal of the mysterious coloring pigment, melanin. Black hair contains concentrated black pigment, while blond hair contains red and yellow pigments. Dark-brown hair has diffused black pigment, and red hair contains red pigments with variations of black or yellow.

Racial characteristics also determine color, thickness and curliness of the hair. American Indians, for example, have long, thick, straight black hair. The Chinese have similar hair, except that theirs tends to be oilier. Blacks have short hair that tends to be very wiry. (It's interesting that these races do not show a serious tendency to baldness.)

The study of hair has turned up many other fascinating bits of knowledge. If you've ever shrieked through a horror movie, you may have seen hair supposedly "growing" on a corpse's scalp. Indeed, it could *look* that way. Upon death, the skin around the hair follicles contracts and draws back, making the hair seem longer by contrast. Actually, since the hair is as much a part of the body as the heart is, its growth stops when the heart stops beating. And can shock turn a man's hair white overnight? Surprisingly, it can (and does). Doctors have observed that extreme emotional stress, such as a shattering battlefield experience in wartime, can cause the pigment granules of the hair to disintegrate with immense speed. When the pigment goes, the hair becomes colorless. White hair, you see, really lacks color, while graying hair does retain some natural pigmentation.

Sometimes young people have a tendency toward prematurely gray hair. What causes it? It's usually the result of a defect in pigment mechanism formation and will most often be found in families where there has been a history of early graying.

Prematurely gray hair is not an especially common problem in your age group. What *is* common is dandruff.

Dandruff is perplexing. Like acne, it can cause distress or embarrassment, but it is not serious or fatal. Dandruff is the most common single ailment of the scalp. Medically it is termed *pityriasis capitis.* Another term for a dandruff condition is *seborrhea.* These terms stand for an abnormal shedding of the scalp in which white scales appear on the hair, hairbrush and comb and on the shoulders of clothing. There are two types of dandruff: *oleosa* or oily, and *sicca* or dry. The type is determined by the amount of oil or sebum secreted by the sebaceous glands. When hair is excessively oily, and won't hold a set or wave, it can become a real embarrassment. The basic causes of dandruff are a faulty diet, emotional tension, hormonal disturbance, infection

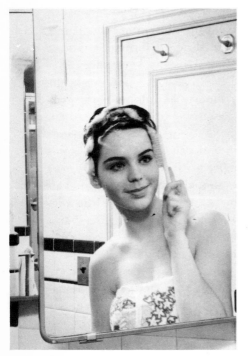

Proper shampooing is one way of combating dandruff, the most common single ailment of the scalp. If your scalp tends to be normal or dry, once-a-week shampooing is fine. If your hair is on the oily side, shampoo twice a week with a detergent shampoo. Massage lather well into the scalp for best results. *(Cleanliness Bureau Photo)*

due to disease, injury to the scalp and unwise or excessive use of hair cosmetics.

Dandruff, along with acne, is seen more in teen-agers than in other age groups. The reason is that during the teen-age years, the body secretes relatively more androgen hormones and so is prone to dandruff conditions.

The foods you eat aggravate dandruff. Too much chocolate, nuts, shellfish, iodized salt, butter and fried foods in the diet increase the skin's production of sebum, which can cause dandruff. Alcohol, too, is a villain.

Emotional tension, which is part and parcel of growing into adulthood, also contributes to dandruff. Exams, dances, competition—anything about which you care very much—can slowly build up tension and cause the nervous system to influence the sebaceous glands to secrete more sebum.

Once in a while, we find that hormonal disturbance can be a major cause of dandruff. Laboratory studies of the surface of the scalp can reveal the presence of bacteria and fungi. This can be treated in most cases with a medicated shampoo or an antiseptic scalp lotion.

If you aren't careful, cosmetics also can cause dandruff. Excessive and careless use of hair spray, permanent wave lotion, bleaches and detergent shampoos contribute to scaling and dryness of the scalp.

Do you have dandruff? If so, here's what you can do to correct it:

1. Shampoo regularly. If the scalp tends to be normal or dry, once-a-week shampooing is sufficient. If hair and scalp are oily, shampoo several times a week. As oiliness decreases, lengthen the amount of time between shampoos. There are dozens and dozens of commercial shampoos on the market today, and we can't attempt to list them all. Those with castile soap and olive oil formulas are generally the mildest because they are natural and neutral. Detergent shampoos clean well, but in some people may cause a slight drying of the scalp.

If the popular brands of shampoos seem unsatisfactory,

medicated shampoos may help. These usually contain selenium sulfide, cadmium sulfide, polythiolate, hexachlorophene, bithionol, resorcinol and sulfursalicylic acid compounds. Some of these antidandruff shampoos include Breck One, Double Danderine, Enden, Fostex, Head and Shoulders, Sebulex, Sebutone, Selsun Blue and Zetar. Additionally, there are other medicated shampoos that can be obtained through a doctor's prescription.

Along with a medicated shampoo, the doctor may recommend extra applications of an antiseborrheic lotion or ointment for the scalp. These contain sulfur, salicylic acid, mild antibiotics and stimulating agents. They are rubbed into the scalp morning and night, after you have parted your hair many times in different areas to expose as large a surface of the scalp as possible to the medication.

Post-shampoo conditioners also help fight dandruff. They deposit a light film on the hair to minimize dandruff, and contain ammonium salts. Some brand names are Dandricide, Rinse Away and Scadan. Helpful hair dressings that contain antidandruff ingredients include Sebucare, Top Brass and ZP-11.

2. Brush and comb your hair carefully and thoroughly. Those one hundred strokes a night your grandmother talks about are not now considered necessary. In fact, some specialists say overbrushing is harmful to the hair and scalp. Brush twenty or thirty strokes to distribute oil along the hair shafts and to remove loose dirt, dandruff and dead cells. Use hairbrushes made of soft, natural bristles rather than synthetics. If hair is wet, don't try to brush it. Instead, gently comb wet hair with a wide, blunt-toothed comb.

3. Use hair cosmetic preparations wisely. Always follow usage directions exactly. And keep in mind that frequent bleaching, teasing, roller curlers, permanent wave lotions, hair straighteners, hair sprays, electric curlers, curling wands and blow dryers are artificial and may be damaging to the hair and scalp if *overused.* (Incidentally, the most expensive and sought-after fashion wigs sold today are made from the hair of European and Oriental women who *never* have exposed their hair to cosmetics!)

4. Observe sensible rules of healthful diet and exercise. Sleep, rest and the foods that provide you with the nutrients essential for good health also contribute to a handsome head of hair and a healthy scalp.

Dandruff, bothersome though it is, is just one hair problem. There are far more serious problems of the hair that can afflict people of any age. Today, we know more than ever before about the causes of these special problems and are constantly developing better, more scientific ways of treating them. We'll consider two of these serious hair problems next.

CHAPTER TEN
PROBLEM HAIR: TOO LITTLE

Adrienne was a very pretty girl of sixteen. She had a trim figure, large and expressive brown eyes and a lovely smile. But when she came into the office, her smile wasn't showing. She took off the scarf that covered her head and we saw why. Her hair was becoming thin on the top of her scalp.

We associate baldness with jolly fat men who tell jokes and seem happy with their hairless lot. That picture is not accurate. Baldness is an increasing affliction of our civilization that strikes both men *and* women, young and old.

Anthropologists, half serious, half joking, forecast that within a hundred years *all* men and women will be bald! Why? On the basis of current cosmetic and biological trends, nutritional deficiencies and pollution of the air, water and food, the human body will not be able to produce sufficient hair covering.

Of special significance to you is the fact that baldness is on the increase among women. From 15 percent to 20 percent of all females past adolescence—and many still in their teens—are afflicted by partial hair thinning or early baldness. Among young men, baldness is also on the increase. We estimate that after puberty, about 80 percent of the male population will suffer hair loss.

Those are the not-so-pleasant facts. Now let's explore the causes more deeply and discuss treatment. For make no mistake about it, many kinds of hair loss and baldness can be treated successfully. A subject that used to be a topic for jokes or personal shame and embarrassment has been recognized as the serious problem it is. There's more hope for its cure than ever before.

The medical term for baldness and/or hair loss is *alopecia* (pronounced al-o-peesh-ya). We have identified six major types of alopecia, as follows:

1. Male pattern type baldness
2. Alopecia areata, alopecia totalis and alopecia universalis
3. Female pattern type baldness
4. Seborrheic alopecia
5. Alopecia due to specific diseases and infections
6. Alopecia following pregnancy

Male pattern type alopecia is in a category all by itself. It affects a large percentage of the male population. Its major cause is hereditary or genetic. For instance, if your grandfather, father and other older male relatives in your family have become bald, chances are you will, too, according to Mendel's Law.

Male pattern baldness also has been linked to increased excretion of male hormone. Dr. J. B. Hamilton of the Downstate Medical Center in Brooklyn demonstrated that the excessive production of the male hormone androgen is the most important factor in the development of pattern baldness in men.

Other causes of male pattern baldness include metabolism disturbances that cause the thyroid to perform its secretion functions improperly, and deficiency of trace minerals in the system, such as copper, zinc and magnesium. Still another cause advanced by Dr. M. Wharton Young of Howard University is that the shape of the head can influence hair growth. Oval-shaped heads, says Dr. Young, have poorer circulation than other shapes, and so have poorer hair growth.

Other contributing factors are dandruff, nutritional disorders, infections of the scalp and scalp injury and body infections and diseases.

What are the ways to treat male pattern baldness? There is a concerted effort going on among hair scientists all over the world to find new and better methods of treatment. Some of them seem promising, but all are still a long way from being available to everyone today.

What can you do now? If you are a young man who is balding, and if there is no special history of baldness in your family, you should have a complete physical examination and laboratory studies. These might indicate that the baldness is a *symptom* of an abnormal physical state. We've seen cases where baldness and loss of hair were due to a low-functioning thyroid, secondary anemia or a heart or kidney disorder. Once the major ailment was diagnosed and treated, the hair loss also was halted and regrowth of the hair was seen.

Emotional tension seems to cause some forms of baldness. It also may cause (through worry over the condition) hair loss to become more serious. Keep in mind, though, that if hair loss is spotty, sudden and rapid, there's a good chance that the lost hair will regrow in several months. If it doesn't, then consult a dermatologist. Your local medical society can recommend a competent specialist in your area.

There also are several methods of disguising male pattern baldness. One is hair transplantation, a surgical technique in which healthy hair roots are taken from a "donor site" where hair is growing normally, and grafted into a bald patch. It is a complicated procedure, averaging about 200 hair grafts per patient, and taking up to six months to achieve new hair growth. It is also not always successful. But it is the only procedure that utilizes your own hair, is a one-time expense and provides results that should last a lifetime.

A second method is hair weaving, in which the patient's own hair is woven or braided to form an anchoring base, into which wig hairs are sewn, woven or knotted. The hair is then trimmed and styled to blend with the natural hair. While it can look well, it needs to be retightened every four to eight weeks as the anchor hairs grow out and shift the woven hair around. This, of course, is a continuing cost. In some cases, the tension created by the tight braiding of the anchor hairs can cause temporary traction alopecia—similar to that caused by ponytails or pigtails.

Thirdly, there is hair implantation, a procedure in which a hairpiece is attached directly to the scalp. First, stitches or other types of anchor points are inserted into the scalp by a physician. Then a hairpiece or tufts of hair are attached to the individual stitches. Although this method provides "instant" hair, it often causes scalp infection and scarring. Since proper cleansing of the scalp is difficult, unpleasant odor also may result. Specialists today consider implantation, therefore, the least desirable solution.

The second major type of baldness comprises *alopecia areata, alopecia totalis* and *alopecia universalis.* Know your Latin? Those three terms refer to patchy, or area baldness, to baldness of the entire scalp, and, finally, to loss of hair on the entire body (eyebrows, eyelashes and body hair). Happily, this type of baldness rarely occurs in teen-agers. When it does, we find it's usually the result of emotional tension combined with some radical change in hormonal secretion. It is characterized by irregular shapes on the scalp that spread and merge. When it does appear in young people, it often cures itself. The returning hair appears first as a downy, colorless fuzz. Eventually, the fuzz returns to natural color, texture and growth.

This distressing type of baldness does respond well to treatment. We have had very good results with the use of hormones like cortisone derivatives (corticosteroid), taken orally and by injection.

Female pattern type baldness is a third type that's of concern to the ladies in our audience. Years ago, a doctor rarely saw cases of female baldness. Today, in the office and clinic, we may see several cases a day! There are many reasons for this unfortunate upswing. In the last century, females had long, healthy hair that was mostly untouched by cosmetics. In the twentieth century

—especially during the last five years—new hairstyles and cosmetic aids designed to improve the "look" of hair have appeared on the market and become enormously popular. And who are the biggest fans for all these new hair cosmetics? Teen-agers. The result is that more young women have more hair problems because of overzealous use of hair cosmetics. *Sensible* use of these cosmetics doesn't cause damage.

The normal growth pattern of the hair is a well-balanced, delicate operation. It is disturbed by unusual pulling or traction upon the hair and the hair bulb—a factor in some current hairstyles. It also is disturbed by the practice of excessive teasing of hair, by daily and overnight use of rollers and curlers. Other villains are cosmetic chemicals used for permanent waving, hair straighteners, hair sprays and lacquers and peroxide bleaches.

Many of the young women like Adrienne who see us about their thinning hair problems plead guilty to these harmful hair practices. We tell them that continuous exposure of the hair to traction and to harmful chemicals definitely disturbs the growth pattern of the hair and may eventually cause the destruction of the biochemical synthesis of the hair.

Serious? Yes! We mean to be. For instance, in a study of twenty-four cases of baldness among young women, Dr. Albert H. Slepyan, a University of Illinois dermatologist, attributed *all* of the cases to continuous use of the ponytail hairstyle. Once the young gals switched from their ponytails to less destructive hairdos, there was regrowth of scalp hair in every case but two.

The first symptom of this type of hair loss is the appearance of red spots on the scalp, combined with scaling or excessive dandruff. The edges of the hairline recede into round or oval bald spots the size of a half dollar. The very same symptoms occur along the front edge of the scalp among girls who have used rollers (especially brush-type rollers) too frequently.

If *you* notice red spots on your scalp, a receding hairline or spotty areas of baldness on your scalp, seek immediate treatment from a dermatologist. He can help you by advising on the hairstyles and preparations that are safest for you, by prescribing medical treatment and by counseling you on the steps for proper hair and scalp hygiene.

Incidentally, Adrienne, who led off this chapter, is progressing nicely. She has changed her hairstyle, is careful about the hair preparations she uses and is watching the food she eats to maintain a balanced diet. This program, combined with the medical treatment we prescribe for her regularly, has started good regrowth of her hair. And in the meantime, she is being very fashionable by using a small wiglet to conceal her hair loss and add glamour and body to her hairstyle while her own hair grows in.

All of which leads us to a brief bit about wigs and hairpieces. Some types of baldness cannot be cured now. We hope that within the next few years they will be. Still other cases require many months to achieve good new hair growth. For these people, wigs, hairpieces and wiglets are a good solution to the problem of appearance. In fact, the embarrassment once associated with wearing a wig has just about vanished. So many prominent people in all walks of life wear them of necessity or by choice that wigs are considered *way in*—fashionable and fun. (You would be amazed, too, at the number of celebrities who wear wigs because they *have* to. And it doesn't seem to bother them one bit.)

In any case, the fashion image of wearing wigs provides you with a big bonus. Never before has there been such a variety of attractive hairpieces so attractively styled in so many price ranges. Hairpieces today look natural, can be cared for, cleaned and styled at home. They are made of different materials. Inexpensive synthetics can be used for fun, for a second hairpiece, or for sports wear or under scarves and hats. Hairpieces made of human hair are much more expensive. Machine-made transformations are less expensive than hand-sewn ones. They are stitched round and round in layers, and therefore look a bit less natural. Hand-sewn wigs look absolutely natural, since they follow the natural hair growth of the scalp, with each bit of hair individually placed into the net base of the wig. The best human hair wigs and hairpieces come from Europe, where the hair has been untouched by damaging cosmetics and is in a glossy, natural condition. Because of the boom of wigs and hairpieces as fashion accessories, wig cleaners, adhesives, wig blocks and other special aids are available everywhere. In choosing a hairpiece for medical purposes, the best idea is to have it fitted personally by a reputable wig manufacturer or salon stylist. He also will advise you on care. A good-quality wig, well styled and fitted, is indistinguishable from the real McCoy. And it can provide you with the important bonuses of self-confidence and poise that are important weapons in conquering your worries about hair loss.

Now let's get back to some of the more unusual causes of hair loss. Seborrheic alopecia also can lead to thinning hair and even baldness. This type of alopecia is caused by excessive oiliness and dandruff. The dandruff, in turn, is caused by overproduction of the sebaceous glands. This condition usually can be corrected by treatment with a medicated, astringent shampoo that will prevent further hair loss as it frees the scalp of dandruff, scaling and itching. Once the condition is corrected, the lost hair will be replaced by new hair growth. In particularly bad cases of seborrheic alopecia, we also recommend close attention to diet. Reducing the body's intake of sugar, starches and fats contributes markedly to an improvement of the hair and scalp condition.

Sometimes seborrheic alopecia in girls indicates a more serious hormonal disturbance. In these cases, the menstrual cycle may be irregular, disrupted or delayed. There may be excessive hair growth on the face, forearms and body. Sometimes there is slow development of the mammary glands of the breast. If these symptoms are apparent in any degree, it's important that the young woman see a doctor. He will advise laboratory studies to examine thyroid secretion; to determine overactivity of the adrenal glands; and occasionally, cytological examination of the cervical tissue to check on estrogen secretion.

Other types of baldness include alopecia resulting from specific diseases, such as pneumonia, scarlet fever, typhoid fever and tuberculosis. Other forms may be caused by viruses, from injury to the scalp and from scalp scars. Some of these diseases and viruses attack the hair shaft and bulb internally and impair circulation. Today, however, with the array of drugs and antibiotics available at our command, these types of baldness can be corrected with proper diagnosis and treatment, and hair loss rarely is permanent. The same is true of hair loss resulting from pregnancy. You can see what a long way we've come in both understanding and treating the various causes of baldness!

But is there anything *you* can do about the subject, as an intelligent and concerned young adult? Indeed there is! Most important to remember is that a healthy scalp and healthy hair require *constant cleanliness.* Cleanliness, all by itself, can combat a variety of diseases. Here is a five-point program to follow:

1. Shampoo regularly. If your hair is dry, shampooing once a week is fine. If your hair and scalp tend toward oiliness, shampoo twice a week. Choose a shampoo that is chemically nonirritating to the scalp. Dry hair requires a shampoo containing oil. Oily hair needs a non-oil-producing detergent shampoo. If you are in doubt, ask your doctor. He can also recommend a prescription shampoo that's just right for you.

2. Comb or brush your hair daily. Never use a stiff nylon-bristle brush! Pointed nylon bristles are too harsh and eventually will injure the scalp. Use a brush made of animal bristles, instead. And choose your comb carefully. It should be sturdy, yet flexible, with rounded teeth that won't abrade the skin or contribute to local scalp infections. Tortoiseshell, while more expensive, is an excellent material for combs. If you do buy a plastic or nylon comb, be very sure that the teeth are not too sharp or pointed.

3. Massage your scalp every day. Use an electric vibrator and/or your fingertips to stroke the scalp. Be careful not to pull or tug at the hair itself.

4. Don't constrict the scalp circulation. As we've already seen, the scalp and hair are nourished by nutrients in the bloodstream. If the blood isn't allowed to circulate properly to the scalp, that isn't helping healthy hair growth, is it? So avoid too-tight hats, headbands, anything that interferes with scalp circulation. And don't wear rollers all day!

5. Eat sensibly. Excessive dandruff or oiliness can be the result of improper diet. Too many fats, starches and carbohydrates should be avoided like the plague. Fad diets are dangerous, too, since they often ignore many of the foods needed to maintain a healthy metabolism. Doctors often recommend low-salt diets for hair health, too. There are many salt-free foods and salt substitutes available today. If your doctor recommends cutting down on salt to promote hair growth, avoid these foods: processed meats, cheeses, shellfish, canned fish, spices, relishes, condiments and ice cream, among others.

So much for our first major hair problem. Now let's get on to the next, which also can cause anguish. It's the problem of too much hair.

CHAPTER ELEVEN
PROBLEM HAIR: TOO MUCH

Munch the peanuts and cotton candy. Watch the elephants and clowns and acrobats. Circuses, as they say, are for "children of all ages!" But along with the glitter and the glamour goes the sad side of the circus—the freaks. You stare at the Fat Man and the Dwarf and the Bearded Lady and you're glad you're you.

The Bearded Lady and the others all suffer from severe glandular disturbances. In fact, too little hair and too much hair both are caused by glandular imbalance, as are dwarfism and giantism.

The problem of unwanted hair can become a real anxiety to females in an age where fashion bares more of the skin. Excessive facial and body hair are not attractive with bare midriff, bikini, sleeveless and strapless styles. Luckily, though, it's a problem that has several practical solutions. Before we discuss them, let's look at the causes of the condition.

Hirsutism is one word for unwanted hair that you may have heard. It is defined as the excessive growth of hair on the face, lips, body, arms and legs. Another term for unwanted hair is *hypertrichosis,* or excessive growth of hair in areas where hair commonly would appear as fuzz. Hypertrichosis is confined to local areas, while hirsutism can be a more general and wider-ranging problem.

We suggested that too much hair is caused by a glandular disturbance. There are several possible causes. In some cases, the pituitary or the adrenal glands, which control hair growth, are out of balance. In other cases, it is the malfunctioning female ovary that causes overproduction of hair as well as other masculine characteristics. A diseased ovary also can cause irregular menstrual periods, underdeveloped breasts and inability to conceive children. This group of symptoms is called a Stein-Levinthal syndrome. In extreme cases where the ovary is found to be diseased, doctors can surgically remove a portion of the ovary and restore the patient to normal body functioning.

Most cases of unwanted hair don't require such drastic procedures! Let's go over the major methods of treatment—both temporary and permanent—and check out their benefits and drawbacks.

1. Plucking away hair with tweezers. This method is probably used most when you want to remove extra hairs from the eyebrows and from between the eyebrows over the bridge of the nose. It can be a safe and harmless way of shaping the brows if you follow these steps:

First, clean the area with alcohol applied to a bit of cotton. Then dunk your tweezers in alcohol to sterilize them before you begin plucking. Use a magnifying mirror and a good, bright overhead light. Cool the area beforehand with an ice cube to minimize the bit of pain you'll feel when you pluck, and wet with a thin line of soapsuds, to soften the hairs. Then, pluck *just a few hairs at a time,* using a quick upward movement. Don't pluck a complete area all at once. It will be more painful and increase the danger of infection. When you are through, apply an antiseptic ointment or a bit of soothing calamine lotion to the area to guard against infection.

There are some other words of caution about plucking away unwanted hair. First of all, hair is not permanently removed by plucking because the papilla is not damaged and will produce a new hair within several weeks. Secondly, the myth that plucking reduces the growth of new hair just isn't true. We've found no

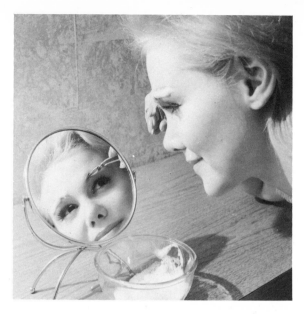

Tweezing is a safe and harmless way of shaping the brows if you observe a few precautions. Clean the area first with alcohol. To make plucking more painless, a coating of soapsuds softens the hairs. Pluck just a few hairs at a time, then apply an antiseptic lotion to guard against infection. *(Cleanliness Bureau Photo)*

medical basis for this belief. And finally (and most importantly), *do not pluck a hair* growing from a wart or mole. You may cause serious bleeding or infection. If an unwanted hair from a growth bothers you, it's better to snip it short or to see a dermatologist about it.

2. Removing hair by shaving it off. Like plucking, shaving does not permanently remove hair. Its advantages are that it's just about painless and easy to do. Its main drawback is that there's a chance of an accidental cut which can cause bleeding and infection. Shaving is mostly used by females for removing underarm hair as well as hair on the arms and legs. (Interestingly enough, our top male swimmers also shave their body hair to reduce resistance to water and increase their swimming speed!) For shaving, follow these simple steps:

First, wet the area and apply a shaving cream to soften the hairs, reduce the possibility of skin irritation and permit closer shaving at the skin surface. Then shave the area with a razor and rinse with warm water. Finish off by applying a soothing body lotion or talcum powder. Or, use an electric shaver that is designed especially for women. Electric shavers work best on hair that is shorter.

Incidentally, we've found no truth in the belief that frequent shaving of the hair causes it to regrow more rapidly.

3. Removing hair by abrasion. This method removes hair temporarily by breaking it off with a rubbing action. You use a pumice stone that fits into your hand. Then you rub the stone onto a small area until the excess hair is rubbed off. Your skin can be moist or dry. Abrasion does not remove the hair too closely to the skin and a stubble will remain. We don't recommend this method for any but the smallest area of skin, nor do we recommend it for repeated use. It is a fairly uncomfortable method and can irritate the skin. If you do use this technique, follow up by using a healing ointment that contains bacitracin or neomycin.

4. Removing hair with wax depilatories. This method is quite popular. If you don't wish to use chemical hair removers, you might want to try it. Its advantage is that it temporarily removes hair *below* the skin surface, so that the hair takes longer to grow back. Its drawback is that it is a very complicated process. Here's how it works:

First, wash the skin to be treated with an antiseptic soap. Dry thoroughly and apply a thin coating of talcum powder. Then melt the wax depilatory in the top of a double boiler. When the wax is warm and easy to spread, yet cool enough to put on the skin, apply it over the skin surface *in the direction of the hair growth* with an applicator or tongue depressor. Next place a strip of muslin or unbleached cloth over the waxed area. As the wax hardens and dries, it fastens onto the cloth. About twenty minutes later, cloth and wax are ready to be pulled off the skin. Do it quickly, pulling *against the direction of the hair growth.* The excess hair comes off with the wax. Then soothe the skin surface and rinse away the rest of the talcum powder with warm soapy water, massage the skin gently and apply an antiseptic lotion or cream.

5. Removing hair with chemical depilatories is probably the best of the *temporary* hair-removal methods. It's less painful and easier than the wax or plucking method, and its effects last longer than the shaving method—about six to eight weeks. Chemical depilatories usually contain barium sulfate or calcium thioglyco-

For smooth shaving of legs and underarms, wet the area first and apply a soapy lather or shaving cream to check skin irritation and permit a closer, smoother shave.

If you use an electric shaver, make sure it is well out of "water range." *(Cleanliness Bureau Photo)* late in a pearly-white cream base. They act by chemically disrupting the keratin in the hair follicle, causing the hair to break off below the skin surface. Chemical depilatories can be used on the arms, legs and underarm areas. Today, many of them can also be used on the face.

How do you use a chemical depilatory? First, test the preparation on the smooth inside surface of your arm. If there is no sign of redness or irritation after thirty minutes, then it's safe to proceed. Begin by thoroughly washing and drying the area to be treated. Apply the chemical with an applicator or tongue depressor and leave it on according to the package directions—usually ten to fifteen minutes. Then wash the area with warm water and soap to remove the hairs, and end by smoothing cold cream or corticosteroid ointment over the area.

6. Removing hair through electrolysis is the most successful and permanent method of removing unwanted hair. It also is the most expensive. We recommend it as a method for young people when there is a serious surplus hair problem that is causing real unhappiness and distress. Here's how electrolysis works:

The electrologist gently inserts a small platinum needle into each hair follicle, guiding it down alongside the hair shaft to the papilla at the base. Then the operator turns on the electric current, which coagulates the hair bulb. Each hair treated this way can then be removed with tweezers or forceps and will not regrow, if the job is properly done.

There are several important facts to know about electrolysis. First, it's essential to go to a competent, licensed electrologist. Skilled operators have developed an exquisite sense of "feel" and know exactly how to remove the hairs without damage. Secondly, there are two kinds of electric current: *galvanic* and *shortwave.* Galvanic current uses an electrochemical reaction, while shortwave works through an internal heat reaction. The galvanic current requires about fifty seconds to remove one hair. The shortwave current takes half a second. Finally, keep in mind that it's almost impossible to remove all the unwanted hair from an area at one session. Usually, the electrologist requires several weeks to thin out the hair gradually until none remains. The process is expensive, but in many cases the self-confidence restored is worth the cost.

Now, what about you young men? Feel kind of neglected? Well, since hair on the face and body is considered to be male plumage, too much hair is not usually considered a man's problem.

However, there are cases when hairs on the face become ingrown. This means that they do not emerge from the follicle to the skin surface, and can cause infection and irritation after shaving. In these instances, electrolysis is used successfully to remove the ingrown hairs and clear up the local infections.

Now, one final word on hair removal before we turn to the next chapter. Some of the methods we've outlined are tricky, others are expensive. An incorrect procedure may cause permanent damage. So before you try out a treatment, check with your parents and ask your pharmacist. If you are doubtful, consult with your physician.

CHAPTER TWELVE
THE DOCTOR ON DYEING

The use of hair-coloring preparations among all age groups, and among both sexes, is a widely accepted practice today. How times have changed! Just a few years ago, it would have been considered improper to deal with the facts about dyeing, tinting and bleaching in a book for teen-agers. Today, we think that the more you know about hair-coloring procedures, the fewer mistakes you are likely to make. And when hair coloring is used with good taste and intelligence, it can highlight and brighten dull, drab hair and also provide an important psychological lift. We don't advise hair color changes, though, without agreement from your parents.

Most people change their hair color because they want to look more attractive. So you must first consider your own natural skin tone, color of eyes and your natural hair color. Any hair-color preparations you select *should complement what you already have.* Usually, hair a few shades lighter than the existing color is more flattering than darker tones. Keep in mind, too, when you study shades on the color chart at the hair salon or the color pictured on a package of home hair coloring, that those colors are applied to pure white hair. So unless your hair is pure white, your normal hair color will *modify* the sample shade on the chart. The way to be sure of your final hair-color result is to follow package directions for strand-testing. That will show exactly how the color will look on your hair.

Now, what about the hair-coloring preparations themselves? We've come a long way, baby, from the days when a coloring job meant just three or four choices—jet black, bright red, brassy gold or platinum. Today there is a whole spectrum of beautiful, subtle shades from which to choose, in a variety of preparations that provide both temporary and fairly permanent color change. In updating this chapter, we turned to Jill Hee, Clairol's Manager of Consumer Relations, who has helpfully added her expertise to our outline of the different types of coloring preparations and how they work. The six major types are:

1. Permanent oxidation dyes and tints
2. Semipermanent dyes
3. Temporary colors
4. Metallic dyes
5. Vegetable dyes
6. Two-step blonding

Oxidation dyes and tints are the most "permanent" hair colorings available, since they actually penetrate the hair shaft. They last until the hair grows out, and usually need redoing in four to six weeks. These also are the most popular products for home application, since they not only color hair quickly, but provide a variety of natural-looking shades. They all work on the principle of a chemical reaction known as oxidation, in which dye mixed with an equal volume of developer immediately before applying acts upon the hair shaft. Most home-use products are applied as "shampoo-in" hair colors. Some are applied with a brush or applicator using the "parting-and-sectioning" technique.

Are there hazards involved? Some people do have a sensitivity that causes an allergic skin reaction. Therefore, the federal Food and Drug Administration warns on product labels that a patch test must be performed twenty-four hours before each application of the dye. A patch test is done simply by applying the dye to the inner surface of the arm or behind the ear with a cotton

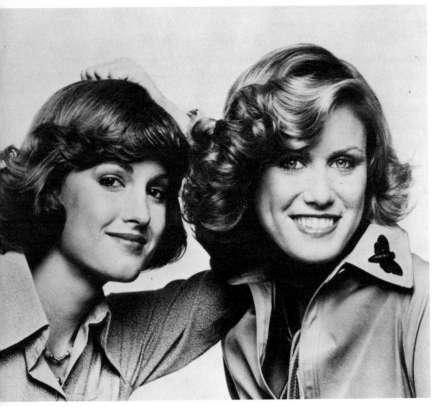

Best friends with two different kinds of hair have used two different hair-coloring techniques to achieve sparkling good looks. At left, "just plain brown" hair acquires rich depths with a semipermanent dye that lasts through several shampoos. At right, lighter brown hair is given golden highlights with an oxidation tint that is shampooed in and will last until the hair grows out (four to six weeks). Remember to perform a patch test for both, and a strand test as called for by package directions. *(Courtesy of Clairol, Inc.)*

swab twenty-four hours before you plan to use the dye on your hair. If no skin irritation develops, then you have no allergic reaction to the dye. If redness, burning, itching or blisters appear, under no circumstances should the dye be used. And a final caution: oxidation dyes should never be used to color eyelashes or eyebrows, because of the possibility of allergic reaction that could cause severe eye damage.

There are dozens and dozens of home oxidation dyes and tints on the market today. Prominent manufacturers are Alberto-Culver, Breck, Clairol, Max Factor, L'Oréal and Revlon.

Semipermanent dyes are dyes that do not require a developer (the oxidizing agent) to color the hair. Therefore, they don't have to be mixed before use. While they produce substantial color change that lasts through several shampoos, they are much less "permanent" than oxidation dyes. They make your own hair color richer or darker, but they will not lighten. (And be sure to strand-test first to preview the color results.) If the dye is left on the hair for the full time indicated on the package directions (up to thirty minutes), then a full coloring effect is achieved immediately. If the dye is left on for a short time (five to ten minutes), then a less noticeable color change occurs. Gradual "small doses" over a period of several weeks can achieve the same strong color change as one large initial application, and this method is good for those who want to be subtle about changing their hair color.

Semipermanent dyes, while considered less sensitizing than oxidation dyes, also require a patch test twenty-four hours ahead of time. (Incidentally, *always* perform the patch test before every new application of dye. There is always the possibility that you may become allergic, even to a product you've used before.) Semipermanent dyes are most effective for small color changes. They also perform well in coloring partially gray hair.

Semipermanent dyes for women are manufactured by Clairol, L'Oréal and Nestlé in rinse, leave-in and aerosol foam forms. Clairol's Great Day is a semipermanent coloring for men.

Temporary colors are designed primarily to add highlights, tone down yellow or gray hair, brighten faded hair and blend streaked hair. They won't produce drastic color changes, and the color is easily removed by shampooing. They contain mild organic acids and are available in either dry or liquid form. In dry form, a small amount of the crystal concentrate is dissolved in warm water and poured through the hair. In liquid form, it is used as a rinse directly from the bottle.

Temporary color products in both types of formulas are produced by Clairol, Nestlé, Noreen and Roux.

Metallic dyes usually contain a lead compound which combines with metallic salts to deposit a colored film along the hair shaft without penetrating it. To change the color of the hair, several applications usually are required, which is why they also are known as "progressive dyes." Contrary to what is believed, they are not "hair-color restorers," since they do not bring back natural hair color, but merely darken it.

While metallic dyes are easy to use at home (most frequently, by men to disguise graying hair) and produce a very gradual color change, they come in a limited number of shades, mostly in the dark-to-intense color range. They do have the advantage of being considered safe to the skin, with little if any allergic reaction. However, you should exercise care to prevent the metallic dye from coming in contact with mucous membranes or skin lesions.

Metallic dyes for home use include Combe's Grecian Formula 16 and Lady Grecian Formula.

Vegetable dyes are the oldest in existence, going back thousands of years. Once these included indigo, camomile, logwood and walnut hull extract. The only vegetable dye used today is *henna,* which consists of the ground-up dried leaves and stems of a shrub found in North Africa and the Middle East. In fact, henna is enjoying quite a vogue today among those who advocate "natural" cosmetics. It is a temporary dye, coating the hair shaft without penetrating it. The intensity of the color varies with the length of application, but it is considered safe to the hair and almost never produces allergic reactions.

Henna can be used in a number of ways. Some stylists are applying neutral henna, mixed with water and egg, to the hair as a shiner and conditioner. Red henna is the most popular. It can

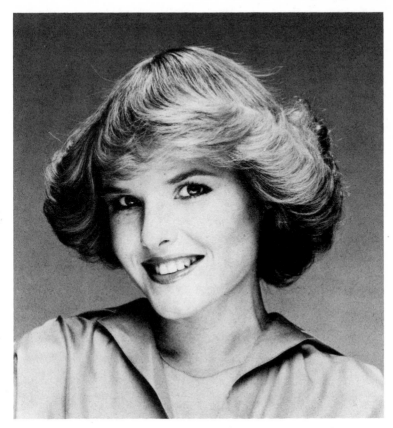

Two-step blonding is the coloring technique used here to lighten the hair several shades. First, bleach is applied, followed by a toner to make the hair exactly the desired shade of blond. This process requires a patch test and the color should always be previewed by strand-testing. It's a technique that should be done by a professional colorist to avoid any hair damage, and it should only be performed on healthy hair that is in good condition. *(Courtesy of Clairol, Inc.)*

be used as an allover rinse, or can be streaked or painted onto the hair, providing red highlights to brown hair, strawberry blond glints to blond hair. Black and brown henna powders also are available. Since results can be uncertain if you do-it-yourself, it's best to have henna applied professionally.

Two-step blonding is a broad category that includes lighteners and toners. The main ingredient is peroxide, and the purpose is to achieve a hair color lighter than the natural shade. Bleaching removes the hair color pigment and provides greater color change than simple tinting. It should only be performed on healthy hair in good condition, since on overcolored or brittle hair it can produce hair damage.

If hair is to be colored two or three shades lighter than your natural color, then pre-bleaching is required. In this process, ammonical hydrogen peroxide is mixed with a hair lightener and applied to the hair to remove color and make the hair fibers more porous. Then the hair is bleached, followed by the use of a toner. A toner may be an oxidation type dye or a nonoxidation type, similar to a semipermanent dye. Toners come in many blond shades, and are applied to bleached hair to make the hair exactly the desired blond shade. The two-step blonding process requires a patch test and the color should always be previewed by strand-testing. We recommend that this process be done by a professional colorist in a reputable salon to avoid any damage to the hair.

Reputable bleach products for home hair lightening are manufactured by Clairol, L'Oréal, Nestlé, Revlon and Roux.

The terms *frosting, streaking* and *hair painting* all describe techniques for bleaching portions of the hair. Frosting is the bleaching of tiny hair strands to add highlights to darker hair. Streaking is the bleaching of broad strands of hair, usually to frame the face. When mild bleach is applied to fine strands of hair with a brush, the process is known as hair painting. These procedures have the advantages of not affecting all of the hair fibers, so regrowth is less noticeable. They also add some body and manageability to the hair.

If you are considering hair coloring for the first time, we advise beginning with small color changes, either with "frosting," semipermanent colors or tints. Both you and your hair are still young, and you don't want to make a mistake. Besides, small changes are easier to do!

If you color your hair, please remember these six pointers for happy results:

1. Don't overexpose color-treated hair to the sun. Some colors oxidize and turn reddish or brassy in the sunlight.

2. Use a neutral shampoo or a special shampoo for color-treated hair.

3. Do not use permanent or semipermanent hair coloring for two weeks before a permanent wave or for one week after a permanent.

4. Be sure to strand-test when you use a new shade, or if you've changed your hair with a permanent or hair straightener. That's the best way to know how the color will look on your hair.

5. Always perform a patch test before each and every application of an oxidation dye, a semipermanent dye or a bleach, even though you may not have exhibited a previous allergic reaction. Metallic dyes, vegetable dyes and temporary rinses do not require a patch test.

6. Try not to change your hair color drastically. A lighter rather than a darker shade is usually most becoming. And plan to style your hair so that you can keep touch-ups about four weeks apart.

Now, let's discuss styling, a subject we suspect is *very* dear to your heart!

CHAPTER THIRTEEN
COIFFURE CARE

Her warm brown hair blown all cloudy-wise about,
Slim as the flags and every whit as fair.
                    —*Lizette Woodworth Reese*

Lively, lovely, healthy hair is a beauty asset. Ever heard of any of these clichés—"pert little redhead," "beautiful blonde," "willowy brunette"? Hair is mentioned so often in songs, poetry and everyday speech because it is one of the first things people notice and remember about you.

A good deal of the attractiveness of hair depends upon the hairstyle you choose and how you care for it. What should a good hairstyle have?

A good hairstyle should suit your size and the shape of your face. A long mane of heavy hair on a petite girl with tiny features looks overpowering, while an extra-short, boyish cut makes a big girl with strong features look even larger. A hairstyle must be in proportion.

A good hairstyle also should look well from all sides—not just the front. Ever seen a girl with an elaborate style that was attractive in front and at the sides, but was a mass of pins and wisps and straggles at the back? Then you know just what we mean.

Finally, a good hairstyle should be easy to manage for your type of hair, and should not need unwise use of hair preparations to keep it in place. As we explained in earlier chapters, excessive use of some hair cosmetics, as well as hair rollers and teasing, can injure your hair and scalp.

Now, let's discuss *you*. Of course, because you are yourself, a unique individual, we can't pick a hairstyle for you. But we can give you some basic rules for choosing a coiffure that's becoming to your size and shape.

In general, tall girls, whether slender or rounded, should balance their height with curved, medium-to-short styles that are full. Long hair should be meticulously well groomed.

Petite figures should scale their hairstyles to their smaller height. Gamin cuts, bubbly and slightly bouffant styles that add a certain amount of height are most flattering, and longer styles should be shoulder-length only.

What about the shape of your face? You should take it into consideration, too. Ideally, the perfect facial shape is oval, and most hairstyles should be planned to give an oval effect. Round faces can be lengthened to ovals by adding top height and through subtracting hair fullness from the sides. Long faces can be shortened to ovals by adding hair fullness at the sides, through wisps of bangs and more body to avoid a droopy look. Square faces can be rounded into ovals through waves and side curls that soften the hair line.

Other special styling tricks for problem features include "lifting" a low forehead with top height, minimizing a large nose by balancing its contours with a bouffant style, getting around glasses by keeping hair away from the forehead and adding fullness over the ears.

The drawback of trying to chart hairstyles for figures and faces is that most of us don't fit easily into a mold. What might be ideal for your best friend might not suit you at all. Suppose you are tall, slightly on the thin side, have a round face and wear glasses. (See what we mean about charts?) In this specific case, we think an away-from-the-face style with a bit of body and back interest would be very attractive. But, as you can see, you have to experiment with different styles until you find one that is most becoming to you. In fact, there are several tricks that can help you. The next time you are shampooing your hair and have built up a good lather, squiggle your sudsy hair into a variety of styles and see which looks prettiest. Maybe it will be most becoming away from your face, or swooshed to one side, or topswept.

Especially attractive for blondes, this casual, yet controlled hairstyle is side-parted and swept away from the brow line. Soft curls at the shoulders are flipped upward here, but can be brushed under for an entirely different look. Electric rollers can be used for a speedy set. *(Courtesy of Clairol, Inc.)*

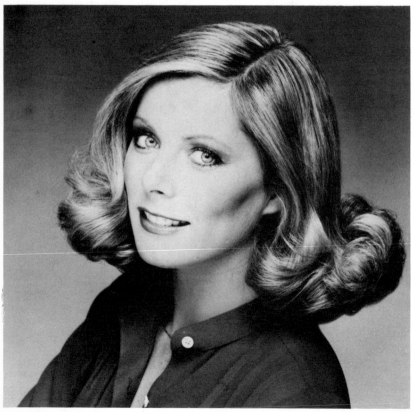

Maybe a side bang or dip would be attractive. It's an easy—and fun—way to experiment.

Another trick to try is to find a full-face snapshot of yourself and ink or crayon out your hair and the photo background. What's left is just your face. What shape is it? Take a piece of tissue paper and draw various hairstyles around your face. Upswept? Full at the sides? Curled under or up? You may hit on a hairstyle you hadn't even thought of!

We said earlier that hairstyles should look well from all sides. The ideal hairstyle is one that is pretty from all angles, with back, front and side interest that flow one into the other. And don't forget the back of your neck. Do you have a pretty, even hairline at the nape of your neck? Or is it ragged and a bit scraggly? Obviously, a raggedy hairline needs concealment, and an even hairline can be accented with a French twist or upsweep.

Perhaps the most important point to consider in coiffure styling is manageability for your own type of hair. The fact is that hair, just like skin, has many individual characteristics. Let's look:

1. Thin, delicate hair. This probably is the kind of hair that Stephen Foster's "Jeannie" had. At its best, it is gossamer-soft, silky and shining. At its worst, it is dry, drab and brittle, and has difficulty keeping a set. Pamper delicate hair with gentle conditioners and shampoos. Hair coloring can give the effect of more body, as can a gentle permanent-plus-conditioners. Avoid any product or process which is harsh on delicate hair, however.

2. Thick, curly hair. This type of hair has many advantages. It can keep a set easily, hold pins, clips and ornaments and can adapt to different styles. However, if it is too thick and curly, it should be thinned and tapered in cutting. If it's cut too short, curly hair can look kinky in damp and humid weather. If too long, it will be hard to style and comb. Extra-large rollers, hair conditioners and setting lotion will keep it smooth and easier to care for. If your hair really is wiry and difficult to handle, you might want to consider hair straightening. (We'll discuss this process in depth later on in this chapter.)

3. Dry, flyaway hair. Baby fine in texture, this hair almost shoots

"Short, sweet and saucy" describes this piquant style, especially good for the petite. Hair is layer-cut all around and tapered neatly at the nape of the neck. It is set on roller curls, then back-brushed for extra height and body. The *guiche* effect at the cheeks is achieved with setting lotion and transparent tape. *(Courtesy of Clairol, Inc.)*

Fine-textured hair goes glamorous when treated to a gentle permanent-plus-conditioners to add body. The layered cut is then set on three tiers of rollers and brushed upward to frame the face. *(Courtesy of Clairol, Inc.)*

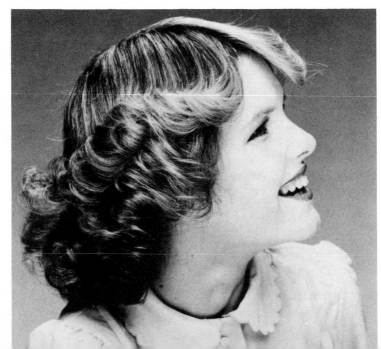

sparks when it's brushed or combed. Dry hair can be caused by an underproduction of sebaceous oils in the scalp, also causing a dry scalp condition. Hair also can become dry from overtreatment: permanent waving, bleaching, tinting and the like. Overexposure to the drying effects of weather also can cause hair to become brittle and dried out. If this is your problem, treat the dry condition with a dry-hair formula shampoo, followed by a creme rinse to reduce static electricity. (Or, before brushing hair, try this trick: rub the hairbrush with an anti-cling sheet that's sold for use in clothes dryers.) A hair-conditioning spray or dressing can be used during the comb-out to add luster and control.

4. Oily hair. Oily hair can be lustrous and vital-looking. On the other hand, it also can look greasy, limp and lackluster. Caused by overproduction of the sebaceous glands, oily hair and scalp should be shampooed at least twice a week with an antidandruff or castile soap shampoo. You may also find it helpful to cover your hairbrush each day with clean gauze that absorbs oils as you brush. Keep your hairstyle one that is easy to manage. Long styles are apt to look limpest when they get oily. A medium, short or upswept coif usually is most flattering.

Those are four basic kinds of hair. Most of us have hair that combines fine and coarse strands. Along the crown and the forehead, for instance, hair is likely to grow more coarsely, while neckline, temple and side hairs are usually finer in texture. The basic texture of your hair helps determine the styling and care your hair requires.

In hairstyling, permanent waving or hair straightening is a first step to give body and control to the hair. Let's study these two processes.

Permanent waving is a process that uses derivatives of an organic thioglycolic acid, mixed in waving solutions with perfume that conceals its unpleasant odor. The chemicals break the natural linkage of the hair's own shape and then rearrange it, mechanically, through curlers. Necessarily, it makes the hair soft and flaccid.

The first permanent, by the way, wasn't pleasant. Perhaps your mother remembers what it was like. Known as a heat wave, it required that the client sit for a long time under an infrared lamp with hundreds of curlers in her hair. Hot and tiring, it produced a frizzy result that was often less attractive than the original look of the hair. But the inventor of the heat wave, the scientist Nessler, had started a whole new trend in coiffure care.

In 1944, a breakthrough in permanent waving began. The invention of the cold wave opened the doors for a whole new kind of hair curling. Available both in home permanents and in salon permanents, the process involved a prior shampoo, then application of a solution containing thioglycolic acid combined with an alkali salt such as ammonia. The solution was put on sections of hair that were wrapped on curlers and left on the hair for twenty to sixty minutes and then rinsed off with a neutralizer—a peroxide or bromate. Depending upon the texture of the hair, the permanent lasted from three to six months.

Today, the cold wave is universal in both home and salon permanents. It has been refined and improved for added safety, ease and beauty. Occasionally, hair damage can occur with permanents—due to an unskilled operator, an allergic reaction or through carelessness in following directions. However, a permanent can be safe and add to attractiveness if you understand the steps involved.

Let's suppose you're going to use a home permanent. You must decide two points: What kind of wave do you want for your hair and what type of curlers?

If you have *hard-to-wave* hair that is straight, baby fine or limp, choose a home permanent with a solution designed for this type of hair. If you have *coarse, naturally curly* hair, hair that is porous from color treatment or hair that has recently been permanent waved, choose an *easy-to-wave* process. If you've never used a home permanent before, and have *normal, noncolor-treated* hair, use regular-strength solution for normal hair.

Next, decide the type of curl you want. The curl isn't determined by the processing time. It's determined by the size of the curling rod you use. Wound on the standard home permanent rods (small, medium and large), the curl will stay until the ends are cut off. Wound on big plastic rods, the wave will last a shorter length of time (two to three months), but will be more natural-looking and easier to handle. Choose rods according to hair texture. Set coarse hair on large rods, baby-fine hair in small strands on medium rods. As a general rule, use large rods at the crown for softness, medium rods at the sides and small rods at the nape of the neck.

Shampoo first to clean hair and gently dry with a towel. When hair is still slightly damp, section off the hair according to the home permanent directions, and wind. Apply the permanent wave lotion one inch from the scalp to the end of the strand and comb the lotion throughout the strand. Use end papers for smooth winding and protection of the hair. Don't pull the hair too taut. Wind it along the curler rod smoothly and evenly. (Too-loose or too-tight winding prevents lotion from penetrating into the hair and may damage it.) Then saturate each curl at the second application, timing carefully for the amount of curl you want. Always make a test curl according to the package directions. When it's time for the neutralizer to be applied, double-check the directions and follow them exactly. Then rinse out hair in tepid water and you're ready to set it in the style of your choice.

Hair straighteners, for girls with too-curly or kinky hair problems, can make hair sleek and manageable. If hair is very dry, overbleached or tinted, *don't try them.* Hair straighteners must be used with great care to avoid damage and hair loss! Best bet: application by a professional hair stylist.

Straighteners combine a base of thioglycolic acid with an alkali such as ammonia salt. Sound like the formula for a permanent wave? You're right. But they produce just the opposite result. First, the hair is shampooed, then the straightening lotion is applied. While the lotion goes to work, the hair is stretched and pulled with a comb. Great care and judgment must be used so that the hair and scalp are not injured by extreme pulling and stretching. A faulty job can cause hair to break and may even cause partial baldness. (Some new processes even skip the combing step altogether.) Next, after the straightened hair has been combed back, it is covered by a tight cap which helps shape the hair. After the straightening process is completed, neutralizer is applied and the hair is carefully rinsed. In some cases, a conditioner is applied to replenish oils. Then the hair is ready for styling. The effects of the treatment will last from three to six months, and the cost may be justified if the hair is really unmanageable. However, we feel it's a process best done by professionals, and then only when the hair to be treated is in good, natural condition.

Shampooed, waved or straightened—now the hair is ready for styling. Hair stylists use three basic terms which you should know: *cut, set* and *comb-out.* These mean, very simply, the way in which your hair is trimmed and shaped, the methods you use to set it into a coiffure and the techniques of combing and brushing the "set" hair into the finished style.

1. The cut. There are two basic cuts used today—the layered cut, which is scissored either in uneven or in graduated layers, and the blunt cut. When done by a professional stylist, a good haircut follows the growth of your hair, keeps a style shapely and manageable and evens out too-thick hair or awkward spots, such as cowlicks.

Layered cuts are thinned, combed and trimmed into layers to permit a wide variety of looks from one cut. They are the most versatile cuts and provide a natural, springy look and the ability to encourage a natural wave and hold a set.

Blunt cuts are all-one-length styles for longer hair that is worn down and smooth. With razor and scissors, the hair is cut while damp, then trimmed and shaped and thinned during combing. This technique gives shape and evenness and is excellent for thick, long or straight hair.

2. The set. The set determines the eventual look of your hair when the coiffure is completed. Setting is a method of curling the hair to a desired shape and pattern. Setting helps make straight hair curlier and gives it body. It also makes curly hair more

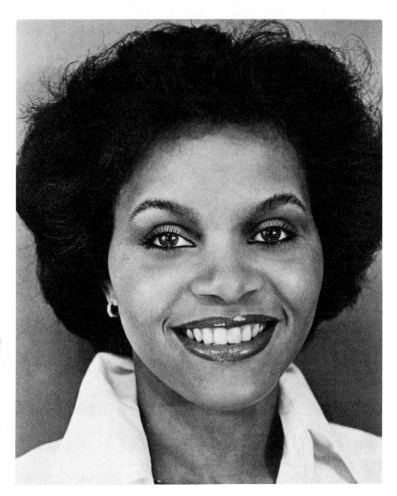

This halo hairstyle is under control. First, hair gets treated to a thorough conditioning, followed by a shampoo. Next, a good cut adds shapeliness, finished off with skillful comb-and-finger styling to "lift" and frame the face. *(Barbizon Agency and School for Models)*

manageable and smoother for a specific hairstyle. All kinds of setting aids are available to help you do a professional hair set at home. And, of course, you can consult a salon stylist for those special occasions.

Let's talk about the variety of hair-set aids available. First, there are *rollers,* probably today's most popular curlers, since they can comb out for a smooth or curly coiffure. Electric rollers have the advantage of working fast, and are very useful for styling hair just before a date. Prolonged use, however, especially on delicate or damaged hair, is not recommended. Other nonelectric rollers are made of plastic, mesh, polyfoam or perforated metal. Use large rollers if you want curves, medium rollers for curlier hair with more bounce and small rollers for fine-textured hair, neckline and tiny curls. Never sleep on rollers all night, though. That can cause excessive tension on hair and scalp and contribute to hair loss.

To use rollers, section off strands of hair slightly narrower than the roller. Comb hair through and wind either away from or toward the scalp. Secure each roller with clips or roller pins, being careful not to wind too tightly—this damages the hair. (Foam rollers, incidentally, produce the least amount of tension on the hair.)

Another new product (actually, an update of an idea used many years ago) is the *electric curling iron* or *curling wand.* This handy little gadget can create curls in seconds, and is excellent for quick touch-ups, provided it is not overused.

Pin-curl clips are used for the wispy hard-to-curl sections of the head: neckline, temples, bangs, as well as for close, tight curls. You secure pin curls either with metal or plastic clips or with bobby pins. You form them as a flat ringlet around your finger, then fasten them flat until they dry. Pin curls can be wound either backward or forward. If you want a wave, you wind one row in one direction. Directly underneath, you wind another row in the opposite direction. Then you comb out both rows in the same direction, emphasizing the wave with your fingers. Stand-up pin curls stick up straight from the scalp and have the advantages of height and bounce. Wind them around your finger just as you do a flat pin curl, but place one end close to the scalp so that the curl stands on end. Slip your finger out and fasten with a clip or bobby pin.

Blow dryers are another excellent styling aid. Many haircuts are specifically designed to be set merely with the fingers and a blow dryer. A recommended method to blow-dry for maximum body is to sit with the head down, hair tossed over the face and brushed forward, with the dryer on a medium setting, and held at least six inches away from the hair. Again, as with any electrical appliance, they should not be *over*used on the hair.

Hair spray is a wonderful way to keep a coiffure from collapsing, to help set hair and to touch up wisps and unruly tendrils. Instead of the sticky shellac sprays and pomades of years ago, we have all types of sprays that help the hair without harm. Most of them contain polyvinylpyrrolidone (PVP), which forms a flexible film on the hair that won't dim the luster or become too stiff and strawlike. Developed during World War II as an emergency plasma extender, PVP is soluble in water. Protein is also used.

Hair sprays are useful in many ways, if you remember some simple rules. Choose the right hair spray for the right job. Some have built-in conditioning agents, such as lanolin or brilliantine, which are good for dry, tinted and bleached hair. Superhold sprays control elaborate styles, subdue flyaway and wiry hair, too. Gentle control is provided by mists that help set hair as they keep a coif in place.

Wave sets can be as simple as water (hair can absorb several times its own bulk), or they can be a conditioning spray or a setting lotion. Lotions and sprays come in different strengths, ranging from easy-to-manage through hard-to-hold formulas. They consist primarily of gums.

Other aids for hair sets include puffy *cotton rolls* to curve the hair without curliness. They can shape a lifted bang or the ends of a pageboy, or give a lift at the temples. *Transparent tape* is a useful aid for shaping *guiche* cheek curls, wispy bangs and forehead curls. Comb damp hair into shape, secure with transparent

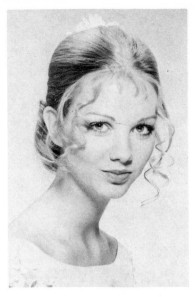

The dress-up look for those of you with longer locks. Perfect for parties, proms and graduations, it features smooth back-brushing from a short center part. The back is arranged in a French twist, outlined here with daisies. Delicate tendrils frame the face. *(Courtesy of Clairol, Inc.)*

The classic pageboy works very well on shorter hair. Here, hair is blunt-cut and bangs are curved to accent expressive eyes. Use large rollers to set bangs and ends. Regular conditioning is a "must" to keep simple styles like this looking their satiny best. *(Courtesy of Clairol, Inc.)*

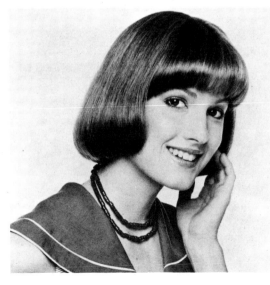

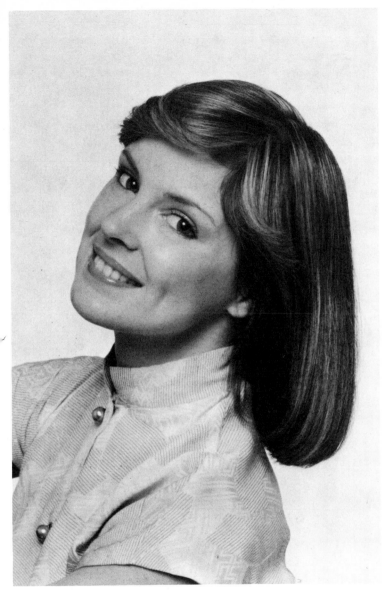

An easy-as-pie hairstyle that starts with a good cut, then is simply maintained by brushing and blow-drying. Subtle frosting adds highlights. The same effect can be achieved by hair painting, in which mild bleach is applied to fine strands of hair with a brush. *(Courtesy of Clairol, Inc.)*

tape until dry, then comb out. *End papers* keep hair ends smoothly in place without bunching or splitting. You'll find them useful with rollers. Buy them or make them yourself out of tissue paper squares. *Bow clips* are pin-curl clips with tiny bows attached. Pretty enough for public view, a few can set a stray curl or two before a date without anyone knowing the difference.

All set? Hope so! Let's move on to the final stage of coiffure care: the *comb-out.* The comb-out determines the final look of your set and it takes a few special tricks to accomplish. Here they are, step by step:

1. When hair is completely dry, remove curlers, rollers, clips. Let the hair rest a few minutes. Then brush hair vigorously with a natural-bristle brush. If you brush in the opposite way from the way you want the finished style, your coiffure will have more "flow" and body, the experts say.

2. Starting at the top, section the hair into its style elements. Arrange each section carefully with comb and brush. Brush top hair into place and complete styling with your fingers to poke and encourage wispy bangs, curls and edges into place. Spray lightly to hold. *Voilà!* As the French say, that's it. You've done it.

Nice? We certainly hope so. Now, let's leave the field to the men for the next chapter.

CHAPTER FOURTEEN
MOSTLY FOR MEN

They sat side by side in the barber shop.
Sandy asked for "a little lift on top."
Pat protested, "That's too much curl."
(Sandy's the male, and Pat's his girl!)
—*B.H.*

Even with the emphasis on unisex hairstyling, too many young men still don't spend enough time on hair and scalp care. Back in Chapter X we outlined basic hair care, which included regular shampooing, careful daily combing and brushing, daily massage for good scalp circulation and sensible eating and exercise habits. A very good reason for doing all this is the fact that after reaching maturity, about 80 percent of the male population will suffer hair loss. And even in your age group, baldness is on the increase.

What does this mean to you personally? We think now is the time for you to start thinking about your head. (Your brain is located there, so it's a convenient place to start.)

We know that a great many disorders of the hair and scalp can be avoided if the scalp is kept clean and healthy. The *clean* scalp will resist a wide variety of diseases and will be a good breeding ground for a healthy crop of hair.

We've already discussed, in detail, the importance of sham-

123

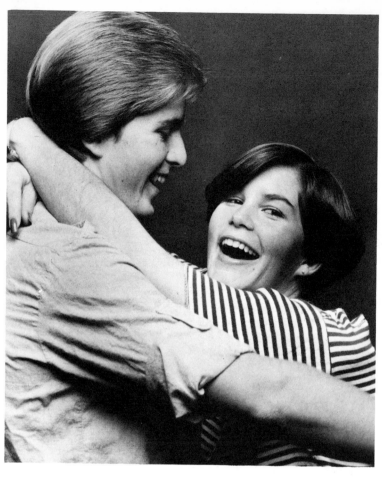

An hour at a unisex hair salon produced these good-looking go-togethers. Regular shampooing and conditioning keeps both his and her hair styles glowing with good looks. *(Photo Courtesy Sebring Products)*

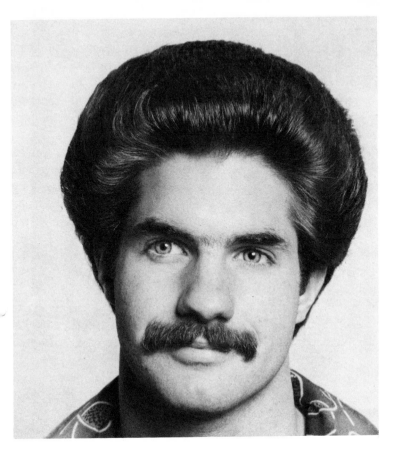

This handsome hairstyle for a husky guy goes from sports to discos looking beautifully groomed. Hair was lightly permed to provide body, then fullness carefully tapered to accent eyes and balance a broad neck and shoulders. (Good styling means a cut that is in proportion with your body as well as your face.) *(American Hairdresser Salon Owner Photo)*

pooing. But it's important to know whether your scalp is oily or dry. If yours is on the dry side, a shampoo containing oil is a good idea. If oily, a detergent shampoo is best, since the detergent has a slight drying effect upon the hair.

Everyday massage is also important. There's a technique to proper massage, just as there's a technique to throwing a spiral forward pass or making a parallel ski turn. Massage should be done with careful stroking of the fingertips or the fatty mound of the palm below the thumb. With the fingertips, massage the forehead, the sides of the scalp and the base of the neck and scalp, taking care not to pull the hair itself. In a barber shop or styling salon, the operator uses an electric vibrator, which is placed on the back of the hand, transferring the electric impulses through the massaging hand. Electric vibrators also are available for home use. If you use a vibrator at home, massage the scalp tissues, not the hair shafts, holding fingers tight against the scalp.

Another important pointer for those of you with dry scalp is the application of mineral or vegetable oils. You see, dry scalps are caused by a reduction of natural oils produced by the sebaceous glands. If those glands aren't producing enough oil, the scalp and hair become dry, itchy and difficult to manage. Vegetable oils, such as olive, sesame, peanut, sunflower or castor oil can be used on the scalp as a dressing, combined with small amounts of solubilized lanolin, such as solubilized isopropyl or acetylated lanolin. Hair dressings containing only alcohol or "greasy kid stuff" aren't good for your hair and scalp. Alcohol preparations have a positive drying effect when used frequently, and greasy preparations cause surface debris to collect on the scalp, mat the hair shafts, obstruct the hair follicles and promote the growth of bacteria.

Now let's discuss styling. The whole history of men's hairstyling is a fascinating one. Long or short, hair has gone through many changes through the centuries. In biblical times, men wore their hair to their shoulders. Through the centuries, monks have shaved their hair into *tonsures,* in which the head is shaven clean with a circular fringe of hair left to grow around it. Even part of English history is distinguished by hairstyles for men. From 1642 to 1648, a bloody civil war was fought in England between the Cavalier followers of King Charles I and the Puritan followers of Oliver Cromwell, in a dispute that began over the king's abolition of Parliament. The Cavaliers wore their hair in long, flowing curls to their shoulders, topped by plumed hats. Cromwell's Puritans, or "Roundheads" as they were called, wore drab garments and had their hair uncurled and neatly cropped, as a sign of protest against the beliefs and policies of the ruling class. Poor King Charles, as you remember, lost the war—and his curly-locked head!

Throughout Europe for several hundred years and during our own American Revolutionary era, men's wigs were high-style. Powdered silvery white, they were often elaborately braided and curled. (A warm, woolly nightcap was part of every fashionable man's wardrobe.) In the nineteenth century, beards and moustaches of all types appeared on men's faces. When a little girl wrote President Lincoln in the midst of our Civil War and suggested he'd look handsomer with a beard, he took her advice and grew one. Many of our other presidents in the nineteenth and early twentieth centuries wore beards and moustaches. In fact, almost every home in America had a moustache cup, which was designed to prevent a moustache from being doused in a cup of hot coffee or tea.

The first half of the twentieth century brought the return of short hair and clean-shaven faces. This innovation had a practical cause: war. Beginning with World War I and reaching its peak in World War II, men wore their hair closely cropped. When an armed force of several million men must be barbered and shaved, the philosophy of "the shorter the better" proved practical. In recent years, long hair has returned, along with sideburns, beards and moustaches. So you see, there truly is "nothing new under the sun."

What's ahead? Well, according to styling experts, the trend is toward the casual but controlled look. What's out? Unkempt, shaggy locks. As we write this, shorter hair is seen more and more often. But length still remains a matter of individual preference.

If you think your hairstyling could stand improvement, check over the following pointers:

1. The key to a good-looking hairstyle is the best cut you can

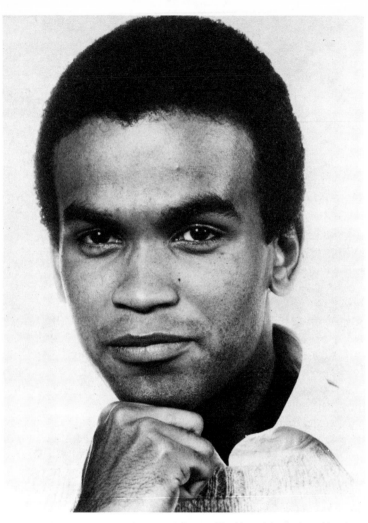

An especially good-looking style designed to show off good bones and features, this short cut depends upon expert scissoring and shaping, looks well for any occasion. To keep it at its best, it needs regular maintenance by your barber, plus regular conditioning before shampooing. *(Barbizon Agency and School for Models)*

get. A good stylist or barber, before he snips a single hair, will study your face, the shape of your head, your overall body height and weight. It is very important, you see, that the hairstyle fit the individual. It must be contoured to fit the head, be balanced and well proportioned. It should also follow the natural growth pattern of the hair. If you have a special problem, such as a cowlick, widow's peak or unruliness, the hairstyle can be shaped to minimize and control these deficiencies.

2. Consider a permanent wave. More and more men are finding that a permanent wave gives their hair body, makes it more manageable and easy to control. A permanent also can provide you with a change of pace in the way you style your hair. For best results, pamper your hair and scalp before having a permanent. For a few days before, avoid vigorous brushing. Use a hair conditioner just before a permanent. As for the type of permanent, select a permanent-plus-conditioner to prevent dry, frizzy ends. After having a permanent, wait a few days before shampooing, and a month before conditioning.

3. Become familiar with the tools of the trade. The stylist uses clippers, shears and razors to cut and trim the hair. Usually, he works from coarse to fine hair when he is working with clippers and shears. If he uses shears and a comb, he cuts over the coarse part of the comb, finishing off over the fine part. For styling, he may use an electric comb, a blow dryer, curling iron or styling brush. Then he may finish off with hair spray to keep the style neatly in place. For your own styling needs, you will find a blow dryer a handy grooming aid, as well as a hair spray. Sprays come in many different formulas, and it is important to pick the one that's best for your own hair and scalp. (Review Chapter XIII for additional information on these "tools of the trade," now used widely by men as well as women.)

4. Black hair care deserves special attention. If you are black, chances are your hair is naturally dry. Therefore, there are certain precautions you should take. Always brush hair gently with a natural-bristle brush. Vigorous brushing may cause breakage. Use a shampoo designed for dry hair, and don't shampoo more

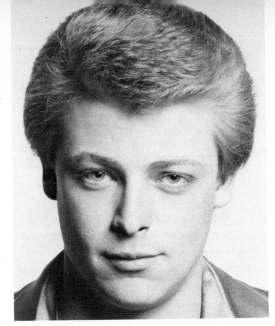

This style is razor-cut to give shapeliness to the head. Easy to maintain, it is styled after shampooing with a blow dryer. Deceptively simple, it is a good example of fine professional cutting. *(American Hairdresser Salon Owner Photo)*

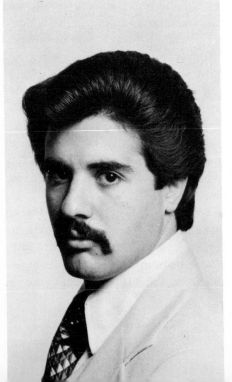

Up-and-away styling follows the natural contours of the hairline, brushed back for a sophisticated look. The fullness on top is planned to balance the moustache, too. If your hair tends to be flyaway, maintain the smooth lines with hairspray. *(American Hairdresser Salon Owner Photo)*

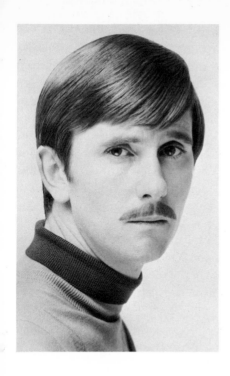

Here's a handsome hairstyle that is smoothly styled by tapering. Keep in mind that a good stylist can eliminate such problems as an uneven hairline or a cowlick by the way the hair is cut. Also note that careful grooming extends to the moustache, which is as neatly trimmed and shaped as the hairstyle. *(Men's Hairstylist Photo)*

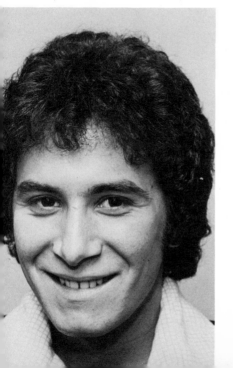

Casually curly, this cut is a good choice to balance a long face and jawline. Here, a permanent adds extra body to a natural curl. Remember, a curly hairstyle must be trimmed regularly to keep it from going "haywire!" *(American Hairdresser Salon Owner Photo)*

often than is really necessary. Don't use blow dryers or electric curling irons often. They can add to increased dryness, brittleness and breakage of the hair shafts. You should also make it a point to condition your hair regularly. Some experts advise deep conditioning every six to eight weeks to keep hair lustrous and healthy. Hair straighteners, for those with too-curly or kinky hair, must be used with great care to prevent serious hair damage. For this reason, we advise having this process performed by a professional. (See Chapter XIII for a full discussion of hair straighteners, too.)

As you can see, there's a lot more to a haircut these days than a bowl and a pair of shears! Hairstyling is a big, booming business and we heartily endorse the idea that a properly styled cut and careful grooming can add greatly to your own good looks.

CHAPTER FIFTEEN

FITNESS: FUN AND GAMES

There's one trend in today's world that is absolutely splendid—the emphasis on fitness! Jogging, skiing, playing tennis, bicycling and exercise are "in." More and more young adults are enjoying fitness as an activity to be shared together. In fact, a recent Gallup poll shows that more than half of all adult Americans exercise regularly.

"Meet me for a two-mile run around the park, and I'll supply a picnic" can be a much more rewarding date than an afternoon at the movies chewing on caramels. And, as one college freshman we know said admiringly, as he watched his girl friend bicycling briskly toward him, "You know, sweat can be sexy!"

The health benefits of exercise are obvious. Muscles become firm and supple, the skin feels elastic and alive, overweight and underweight problems are helped, posture is improved, even your brain is refreshed. The vitality that exercise affords is the most modern form of sex appeal.

Of course, as with most everything in this world, there are do's and don'ts in achieving fitness. Trying to overdo without the proper preparation can be damaging. And there are some sports that are better suited to certain body types than others. So let's take a closer look and provide you with some suggestions gathered from experts.

First, exercise requires muscle power. Where does it come from? The energy you need for exercise is supplied within your muscle cells by fats, carbohydrates and proteins. These nutrients, when digested, are broken down and sent to the cells by the circulatory system. They produce a substance called ATP (adenosine triphosphate), which supplies the body with a quick-energy power system. Your muscles have enough ATP stored in them to run a 100-yard dash without taking a breath. Of course, your body can't continue long at that pace, so a backup compound called CP (creatine phosphate) combines with ATP to keep supplying the energy needed for sustained exercise.

You may have heard some sports described as *aerobic,* others an *anaerobic.* The immediate quick burst of energy (ATP) is anaerobic, while the long-term energy system (CP combined with ATP) is known as aerobic, explains Dr. Frank I. Katch in a recent article on body energy. Take jogging for example. Let's say you want to jog two miles along a beach. In the first few seconds, that immediate burst of anaerobic ATP sends you flying. When it runs out, it becomes recharged through the CP reservoir. Then the long-term aerobic system goes into action to supply the energy needed to complete the run. As you get about 70 percent of the way down the beach, you have to slow down. That's where pacing and preparation are important in permitting you to complete the run. Preparation includes exercises designed to improve your body for a specific sports activity. Let's take a look at some of the most popular recreational sports and see how you can get the maximum benefit from them.

As Dr. John L. Marshall, Director of Sports Medicine at the Hospital for Special Surgery in New York City says, "The key is not to play to get in shape, but to get in shape to play." (And even if you are not sports-minded, we do recommend the exercises in any case!)

JOGGING AND RUNNING

Twenty-three million Americans are jogging and running today, ticking off a total of 17 billion miles a year. (That's the equivalent of ninety times to the sun and back.) What's the difference between the two? Generally, runners can do the mile in eight and a half minutes or less, while joggers take a more leisurely pace. The posture in jogging is more upright, with arms high, feet slapping the ground. Running is done in a more slanted posture, with long fluid strides, arms swinging freely, with momentum carrying the weight forward. It's the loose-jointed body types who are often better suited to the endurance or distance sports like jogging and running. The benefits provided by jogging and running are flexibility, stamina and strength. For many, running provides the incentive to stop smoking, drinking and overeating. What are the drawbacks? Runners are especially prone to injuries of the Achilles tendon and knees, and to leg cramps. Those with heart problems and diabetes should check with their doctor before attempting running or jogging. And before you hit the trail, get your body in shape. Here are three exercises that are especially helpful:

1. Slow stretch. Hold onto a railing or table with both hands, and rise up on your toes. Slowly do a deep-knee bend, hold for a count of three, then straighten up again and lower your heels to the ground. Repeat. This stretches thighs, calves and feet, builds up back muscles and improves posture.

2. Bend and twist. Sit down on the floor, back straight, legs apart, arms straight over your head. Bend your body to your right foot and try to touch your head to your right knee. Bounce three times. Then twist toward the inside of your right leg, and bounce three times. Return to starting position. Then switch to the left side and repeat on the inside and outside of your left leg. Do the exercise five times on each side. This is good for the back and hamstring muscles.

3. Stamina shapeup. With legs straight, bend down and place hands flat on the floor. Keeping legs as straight as possible, walk forward on hands until the body is almost parallel with the floor. Pause for a count of three, then walk backwards on your hands until they meet your feet. Repeat four times. This is a great allover exercise that strengthens calves and is easier than push-ups, especially for women.

TENNIS, SQUASH AND OTHER RACQUET SPORTS

These sports require less sustained stamina and physical strength than running and jogging, and are known as anaerobic or "explosive" sports, as they require quick bursts of energy and fast reflexes of mind and body. Since they are *unilateral,* meaning that they use major muscle groups on only one side of the body, flexibility and equal distribution of weight and muscle tone are very important. Ailments associated with racquet sports are tendonitis and back trouble, so here are some exercises to help prevent these problems that should be done as pre-game warm-ups:

1. Jumping jacks. Do this with your tennis partner. Face each other and hold hands to aid balance. Jump together continuously for thirty seconds, landing lightly on the balls of your feet. There's no need to jump higher than an inch or so—the way you land is more important than the height you achieve. This exercise is a good stretcher and strengthener.

2. Side stretcher. Plant feet firmly together. Holding onto a railing or counter edge with one hand, lean away as far as you can, extending your free arm gracefully over your head. Repeat five times on each side. This activates the side muscles on both sides of your body.

3. Shoulder flex. Sit on the floor in a cross-legged position with back straight. Interlock your fingers behind your back, resting palms on the floor. Pull shoulders together by lifting and stretching arms upward. Drop arms and slump forward. Return to starting position and do five times. This exercise shapes up shoulder muscles and eases shoulder tension.

HIKING AND BACKPACKING

If you are an outdoors-lover, these sports are especially good. They span the seasons, are a great group activity, and can be done at any pace you set. Similar to jogging and running in their long-range endurance requirements, they increase body stamina and strengthen the long muscles of the body (back, arms, thighs, calves). Problems to watch for are muscle strain, ankle sprains and strains. Asthmatics and those with heart trouble should undertake these activities only after getting a doctor's okay. Here are some helpful preparation exercises:

1. Squat kick. Stand up straight, holding onto the back of a chair with the left hand. Place right hand on waist. Lower your body into a squat position, then raise the body quickly, kicking right leg as high as possible as you do so. Repeat five times. Switch position and repeat five times, kicking with the left leg. This builds stamina and strengthens lower back and thigh muscles.

2. Back-press push. Lie on the floor with knees bent and feet flat on floor. Press lower back flat against the floor. Place hands in back of your head and raise the upper part of your body until shoulder blades clear the floor. Repeat the exercise several times to strengthen the abdomen and back.

3. Push-pull. This is another twosome exercise. Stand facing your partner, who extends arms straight in front toward you. Clasp partner's hands and push partner's arms back and forth in a bending-then-straightening motion. Do this for a minute, then reverse roles, with you extending your arms, your partner doing the pushing. This tones and strengthens arm muscles.

SWIMMING

This is another good all-year-round sport, since most everyone has access to a pool somewhere. It requires average strength and stamina, while providing the benefits of good muscle strength and flexibility. Incidentally, if calories are a concern, doing the backstroke burns off 560 calories in an hour; the sidestroke, 408; treading water, 210 calories. And our grandmothers firmly believed that doing the breaststroke beautified the bosom! Try these warm-up exercises first:

1. Swan swoop. Lie flat on the floor on your stomach with hands stretched out over your head. Have a friend sit gently on your calves. Swing both arms out to the side slowly, and simultaneously lift the upper body off the floor in a 1-2-3-4 count, arching the back. Lower the body back flat to the same count. Repeat four times. This exercise, also good for divers, by the way, arches the back muscles and loosens chest and arm muscles.

2. Flutter kick. This exercise is done best on the edge of a bed. Lie on your stomach, arms tucked under chin, with legs extending straight out from bed. Flutter-kick your legs from the hips, just as you would in the water. This exercise should start with just a minute or so of kicks, gradually working up to more. It strengthens legs, backs of thighs and buttocks.

3. Hip trip. Holding onto a table edge or porch railing with your right hand, stand with one leg behind the other, left arm outstretched. Kick as high as you can with your back (left) leg, then with your front (right) leg. Switch sides, holding on with your left hand, and repeat. This exercise is designed to mobilize hips and buttocks, strengthen inner thighs.

SKIING

In its various forms of downhill and cross-country snow-skiing, as well as water-skiing, skiing is beloved by people of all ages all over the world. It truly is an international sport. While it does require instruction, only average muscle power and stamina are required. Good health benefits are gained in terms of muscular strength and coordination. Hazards to health include sprains, strains, broken bones (particularly if you attempt to ski beyond your level of skill or stamina) and skin damage caused by weather exposure. It is particularly important for skiers to prepare ahead of time with helpful exercises. You must be able to control your skis and not vice versa!

1. Crossovers. Lie on your back, arms out to the side, with chest and ribs up, chin level. Keeping your hips on the floor and pointing your toes, lift left leg straight up. Keeping both legs straight, stretch the lifted left leg over the right hip, turning your head in the opposite direction. Stretch as far as possible. Then repeat with the other leg. This exercise stretches leg muscles, firms waist and thighs.

2. Leg lift. Sit in a straight-back chair. Stretch legs straight out, toes up to ceiling. Hold that position for thirty seconds. (Try to increase by thirty seconds each day.) To add effectiveness to the exercise, wear your ski boots or ankle weights when you perform it. It is a fine means of strengthening upper legs and knees.

3. Knee bends. Stand with your back flat against the wall, with feet placed flat on the floor about twelve inches away from the wall. Lower your body slowly, bending your knees until thighs are parallel to the floor. Repeat several times. This exercise effectively strengthens thighs and upper legs, and is especially recommended for water-skiers.

BICYCLING

This is a fine form of exercise for all body types as well as a nonpolluting means of transportation! Racing cycling is similar to the racquet sports in requiring sharps bursts of anaerobic energy, while cycling several miles at a leisurely pace is aerobic, similar to skiing or jogging. Bicycling, while it requires only average physical stamina or strength, builds and firms the long muscles of the body (arms, back, calves, thighs). Ailments incurred most often by bikers include cramping and muscle pulls, so preparation exercises are a good idea, particularly if you plan a long-distance cycling tour or a visit to the Netherlands, where everyone cycles! Try these:

1. Arch press. This one takes two people. Get down on your hands and knees. As you raise your back to an arched position, have your partner place hands on your back and push down, trying to prevent you from raising it. Repeat several times. Then do the same with your partner, reversing roles. This is a fine exercise for the lower back, and is excellent for horseback riders, too.

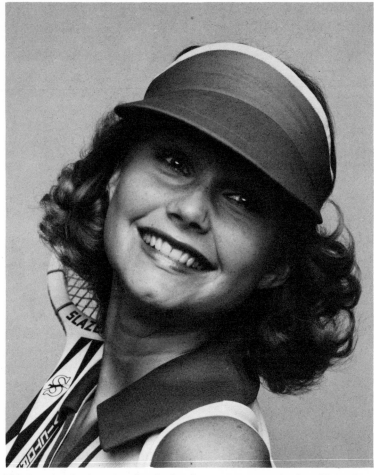

This teen tennis player is a "pro" when it comes to protecting her skin against sun damage. She wears a visor to shield eyes from glare, applies a sunscreen on face, neck and shoulders and protects lips from chapping with glosser, Vaseline or Chapstick. After tennis, she applies an allover moisturizer to keep skin soft and smooth. *(Courtesy of Clairol, Inc.)*

2. Flex lunge. Squat on your left leg, with right leg stretched out to the side. Rest the right leg on the heel, with toe pointing up.

Bounce gently eight times, flexing the foot of the right leg hard, pulling toes toward body. Reverse legs and repeat. Do four times on each leg. This works to stretch legs, thighs and calves.

3. Pony prance. Standing straight, put your weight on the right leg, with your right heel flat on the floor. Lift the left knee straight in front of the body, then lower the left foot to the floor, touching first with toes, then the ball of the foot and finally the heel. Continue doing this in a quick, prancing motion ten times. Then repeat the exercise with the right leg. This strengthens and flexes both the foot and the calf muscles.

So much for some specifics of recreational sports and exercise. Now let's take a look at other aspects of the sporting life you will encounter.

The first is *skin protection.* Skiers, even more than sunbathers, are prone to damaged skin, as the higher the mountain, the stronger the sun's ultraviolet rays become. Snow also acts as a reflector, so skiers get a double dose from both above and below. Therefore, both sexes need extra protection to prevent drying and chapping and eventual skin damage. In addition to reviewing the pointers outlined in Chapter V, you should always use a sunscreen preparation on your face and neck, add an extra protective coating on your nose, lips, ears and neck and protect your eyes and the extrasensitive skin around the eyes by wearing sunglasses or goggles. After skiing, apply an allover body moisturizer or intensive skin care lotion, or bathe in a dry-skin bath oil product. And gals, skiing is one time when you should use a foundation makeup *under* your sun lotion, because of the extra protection it provides.

Hikers, bikers, backpackers and joggers will also need to take special protection against heat exhaustion, insect bites and stings and poisonous plants. We suggest you reread Chapter IV, keeping in mind that your gear should contain insect repellent, an anti-itch cream or gel if the bugs do get you, foil-wrapped towelettes and an all-purpose product such as Vaseline in a tube, which soothes irritated skin, protects lips and moisturizes, too.

A second aspect is *equipment*. We can't stress enough the importance of proper footwear for the sports discussed above. (Remember, your feet are the sole support of your body weight!) Runners, joggers and tennis players must wear well-fitted shoes and socks. For runners, the recommended styles are those with a thick, solid sole, thicker and slightly raised at the heel. Tennis players should be sure their shoes provide good arch support. All sports shoes and ski boots should be wide and roomy at the toes. Ski and hiking boots must provide firm ankle support, as well. For sports requiring socks, two lightweight pairs are preferable to one heavy pair. (Look over Chapter VIII again for specific foot-care pointers.)

As for the rest of the gear you need for a particular sport —apart from essentials such as racquets, skis, bikes, footwear— don't be beguiled by expensive specialized clothing suggested by garment manufacturers. You can function nicely in regular jeans, shorts, tee shirts and sweaters. A basic principle to remember, though, is that in almost every sport outlined above, several lightweight layers of clothing are preferable to one heavy layer. This is particularly true for skiers, hikers and backpackers. Layers are easy to shed or add as you need them, and also maintain the body temperature more effectively.

The third aspect is *pain*. We've already discussed the problems of heat exhaustion in Chapter V, and insect bites, stings and poisonous plants are outlined in Chapter IV. The other common causes of sports-related discomfort are:

1. Cramps, which occur when a muscle contracts and won't relax. The result can be an excrutiatingly painful knot that cripples the runner, jogger or biker. The best thing you can do for a cramp is to stop the exercise, and gently massage and stretch the cramped area. This procedure will relax the knot and permit proper circulation to return.

2. Sore, stiff muscles can occur in any sport, most particularly if no preparation exercises or warm-ups have been performed. That's why advance exercises are so important in the overall fitness picture. However, most minor aches and pains benefit from application of heat. Very painful and tender aches and pains require rest, ice, compression and elevation. If you're not sure, application of ice is a safe bet, since ice acts as an analgesic by reducing pain, constricting swollen blood vessels and minimizing swelling.

To sum up the "message" of this chapter, we quote Dr. Willibald Nagler, Chairman of the Department of Physical Medicine and Rehabilitation at New York Hospital-Cornell Medical Center: "I don't think in the long run it matters very much whether one gets engaged in very fashionable exercises or not. It is much more important to get yourself engaged in some activity in which you are really interested and which you enjoy that has some health value. It is the *regularity* and *frequency* of a physical activity that brings the health and body-shaping benefits."

Now of course, enjoyment of exercise and sports requires fuel—those carbohydrates, fats and proteins that supply the muscle power. Which brings us to the next chapter. Aren't you getting hungry about now?

CHAPTER SIXTEEN
FOOD FOR THOUGHT

Canary-birds feed on sugar and seed,
Parrots have crackers to crunch;
And as for the poodles, they tell me the noodles
Have chicken and cream for their lunch.
But there's never a question
About my digestion—
Anything does for me!

—*Charles Edward Carryl*

How about you? Is "anything" your food philosophy, too? The energy and muscle power needed for the sports and exercise we discussed in the last chapter depend upon a sensible combination of vitamins, minerals, fats, carbohydrates and proteins obtained from the food you eat.

What happens when you've eaten a meal? Very briefly, when food enters the alimentary tract, gastrointestinal enzymes act on the food, digesting it into its specific components, which next are absorbed and then utilized by the body for specific functions and purposes. Here are those components and what they do for the body:

Proteins are the basic material of each body cell. They are the constituents of the muscles, sinews and lean tissues of the body.

144

You need them in your diet to develop tissue, maintain tissue and repair it. Protein-rich foods include eggs, milk, cheese, meats, fish, poultry, beans, grains, cereals and nuts.

Carbohydrates, composed of starches and sugars, serve as sources of energy for the body. Because they are the most economical sources of energy, they are the foundation of most diets everywhere in the world. However, when more carbohydrates are eaten than can be converted into energy, those extra starches and sugars turn into excess body fat. Desirable carbohydrates are found in cereals and cereal products, potatoes, bread, rice, noodles, fruits and vegetables. They also are found in sugar, jams, jellies, candy, soft drinks, honey and salad dressings.

Fats are a rich source of food energy that forms the lipoid tissues of the body. Fats are found in fatty meats, butter, margarine, cream, most cheeses, whole milk, shortenings, mayonnaise and salad dressings, egg yolks, nuts and peanut butter. Because they have a very high caloric value, fatty foods contribute to overweight unless they are assimilated by the body in exercise.

Minerals help form the hard tissues of the body, such as bones and teeth. They also contribute to the proper functioning of muscles, nerves and the heart and help the formation and function of the red blood cells. Altogether, about fifteen different mineral elements are needed by the body. A balanced diet provides the necessary minerals you need. Three of the most important minerals are *calcium* (for healthy blood, bones and teeth), found in milk products, shellfish, egg yolks, nuts, whole wheat and green vegetables; *iron* (for red blood cells and healthy skin), found in organ meats (liver, heart, kidneys), shellfish, green vegetables, lean meats, egg yolks, beans, dried fruits, nuts and wholegrain cereals; and *fluoride* (for blood, bones and teeth), found in milk, egg yolks, oysters, cabbage, mineral water and whole wheat.

Finally, **vitamins** are the essential compounds needed by the body for healthy overall functioning. Since the body does not manufacture its own vitamins, it must obtain them from food. (Or, when prescribed by a doctor, from vitamin supplements.) If your diet is proper, you shouldn't need vitamin supplements.

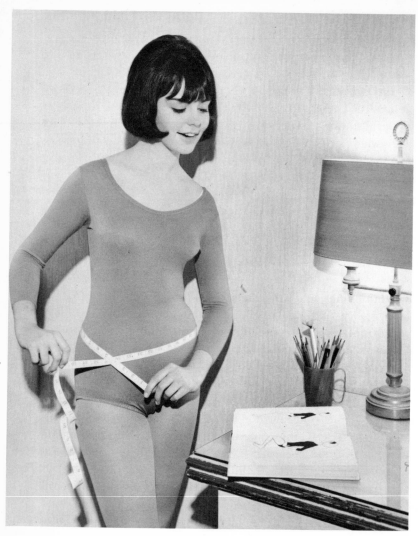

Overweight, underweight or just right? Your weight and figure are related to the calories supplied to your body. A balanced diet of foods selected from the five basic food groups, combined with plenty of daily exercise and sleep, can go a long way in achieving good looks and good health. *(Cleanliness Bureau Photo)*

Often, they are a waste of money. The American Medical Association estimates that $500 million is spent each year by Americans on unprescribed and unnecessary vitamin supplements and diets.

There are two kinds of vitamins: fat-soluble and water-soluble. The chart on pages 148–150 outlines their function and importance to good health.

Now let's talk about food itself. After reading through the food components we've outlined, you may have the feeling that you should eat nothing but liver and egg yolks! That's not the case, of course. Most of the foods we eat every day consist of combinations of the essential diet elements. But there is no one "perfect" food that supplies all our health requirements. For good nutrition and good health, all the elements must work together in a well-chosen variety of foods. There are five basic groups:

1. Milk products group
2. Meat, fish and poultry group
3. Bread-cereal group
4. Vegetable-fruit group
5. Fats and oils group

Good nutrition means that you must eat *some food from each of these groups every day* for good health. That's why the fad diets (grapefruit diet, banana diet, brown rice diet) can't supply all the nutrients you need and can be downright dangerous over a period of time, especially for twelve-to twenty-year-olds whose bodies are still developing. Dr. Frederick J. Stare, head of Harvard University's Department of Nutrition, puts it very well. He says, "Variety is the keystone to good nutrition to develop the best body your genetic potential will permit."

What's the best way to assure you get enough variety and the right foods into your system? For young adults, whose busy schedules usually include a pickup lunch and lots of snacks, the answer is difficult. So, after consulting a good many experts, we reached the conclusion that there are *two* right approaches. We

FAT-SOLUBLE VITAMINS	BODY NEED	FOOD SOURCES	DEFICIENCY/DISEASE
Vitamin A	External tissues of the body, including skin and mucous membrane; needed for night vision; often prescribed for skin conditions, such as acne, to help regenerate skin	Liver, egg yolks, green, yellow and orange vegetables, fish liver oils, milk products	Night blindness, skin problems such as acne (*Note:* too much vitamin A may cause hair loss and dry skin.)
Vitamin D	Bones and teeth; provides needed balance of calcium and phosphorous	Liver, egg yolks, fish, fish oils, milk products, green leafy vegetables, Vitamin D-fortified milk; also manufactured by the skin during exposure to the sun's rays	Rickets (softening of the leg bones), tooth decay
Vitamin E	Reproductive system, muscle tissue and the vascular system; often prescribed for menstrual, menopausal and blood vessel disorders	Whole-grain cereals, green leafy vegetables, suet, organ meats (liver, heart, kidneys)	Dysfunction of the reproductive and vascular (blood vessel) systems

Vitamins F and K	Ability of the blood to clot, thus preventing continuous bleeding	Bran, liver, cabbage, cauliflower, carrots, egg yolks, rice, soybean oil, tomatoes	Hemorrhaging under the skin
WATER-SOLUBLE VITAMINS			
Vitamin B$_1$ (thiamine)	Normal growth, muscle contraction, heart, appetite, circulation, digestion, nervous system	Poultry, fish, pork, organ meats (liver, heart, kidneys), whole-grain or enriched breads and cereals, peas, beans, nuts, eggs	Beri beri (disease producing general debility and rigidity), nervous tension, poor circulation, poor muscle tone
Vitamin B$_2$ (riboflavin)	Transportation of oxygen from one part of the body to another; metabolism of soft tissues, including eyes and skin	Milk products, eggs, lean meats, green leafy vegetables, enriched breads and cereals, dried peas and beans	Eye disorders, cracking of lips, susceptibility to infection, premature aging, loss of weight

WATER-SOLUBLE VITAMINS	BODY NEED	FOOD SOURCES	DEFICIENCY/DISEASE
Niacin (a B-complex vitamin)	Liver, skin, and nervous system; assimilation of carbohydrates	Organ meats, eggs, cheese, citrus fruits, fish, whole-grain or enriched breads and cereals, dried peas and beans, nuts, peanut butter	Pellegra (swelling of the gums and tissues of the tongue), headaches, sleeplessness
Vitamin B_6 (pyridoxine)	Normal growth, hair and skin	Egg yolks, wheat germ, whole-grain cereals, milk, meat, cabbage, fish	Impaired growth, sleeplessness, nausea, difficulties in walking
Vitamin B_{12} (cyanocobalamin)	Blood; often prescribed as a treatment for pernicious anemia	Liver, organ meats, fish, oysters, hard cheese, milk	Anemia
Vitamin C (ascorbic acid)	Teeth and bones, tissue growth, body cells, healing of wounds	Citrus fruits and juices, strawberries, cantaloupe, green vegetables, tomatoes, potatoes	Scurvy (a hemorrhaging disease of skin and membranes), colds and infections, tooth decay, gum disease

suggest you choose the one that suits your own life-style and temperament best.

1. The traditional trio: Three square meals a day, beginning with a breakfast that provides one-fourth of the daily calorie requirements and one-third of the daily protein need. Many food scientists say that breakfast (the meal you're most likely to skip) is the most important meal of the day. An inadequate breakfast leads to a low blood-sugar level during the morning, while a nourishing breakfast aids mental alertness and allows the body to operate at maximum physical efficiency throughout the morning hours. Yet a nationwide study of teen-age breakfast habits showed that 48 percent skip or skimp on breakfast. Perhaps one reason is sheer dullness. But you don't *have* to eat the same old thing every morning. Try different juices and fruits, a variety of hot and cold cereals, unusual ways of preparing eggs and meats. A slice of melon topped with a scoop of yogurt or sour cream, shirred eggs, buttered raisin-bran muffins and a cup of cocoa is a delicious breakfast that is just as nutritionally correct as orange juice, cereal and milk. We believe that if you have a more varied menu at breakfast time, you're more likely to enjoy (and eat) it. The Australians, for example, have always been noted for their substantial breakfasts, which include, in addition to hot cereal, hot meat and potatoes. The English enjoy such hearty fare as grilled kidneys, kippers and lamb chops for their morning meal.

Now we come to lunch. That is probably the most difficult meal to control. While the trend in school and campus cafeterias seems headed in the healthy direction of providing good-quality carbohydrates in the form of fresh fruits and vegetables, some cafeteria food features starchy and dull macaroni and spaghetti menus. So students skip those offerings and munch instead on french fries, hot dogs, soft drinks and candy bars. That kind of lunch is perfectly all right once in a while, as long as you make up for its deficiency with other well-balanced meals and snacks that same day. Or you can, of course, do what is becoming increasingly popular—"brown-bag it" with your own choice of tasty lunchtime foods.

As for dinner, it is important because in many families it is the only meal of the day that is shared. But keep in mind that it needn't be the heavy meal that most Americans eat. In fact, it's better if it is not, since it is difficult for the body to digest and absorb all that food properly before bedtime. (In many parts of rural America, the noon meal is the most substantial, providing energy for the afternoon and early evening hours.) Harvard's Dr. Stare adds another caution, saying, "If you go out to some steak house where they brag about steaks that are twelve ounces, it's too much. You ought to eat about three or four ounces of steak."

2. Scientific snacking: Five small meals spaced throughout the day, to keep energy up. This "scientific snacking," according to home economist Ellen Katz (herself pretty and slender), is ideally suited to a young adult's life-style and can provide all the necessary foods you need in amounts that are quickly digested and utilized by the body. "Our stomachs have no clocks," says Mrs. Katz, but they must be fed and nourished. So she suggests (1) a well-balanced breakfast, (2) a light lunch, (3) a midafternoon snack, (4) a light evening meal, and (5) a midevening snack. She explains that each of these smaller meals provides greater opportunity for you to eat foods from each of the five basic food groups without "overloading your body."

We don't have the space in this chapter to cover entire menu plans or give recipes, but to illustrate the "snack" concept of eating, here are some nutritious snacking ideas:

1. Dippy vegetables. Raw vegetables contain a wealth of nutrients, but many people find them boring all by themselves. So create a dip that perks them up and turns them into a treat. The simplest one is yogurt with a squeeze of fresh lemon or lime juice. Chill, then dunk. Or combine equal parts of mayonnaise and yogurt and season with dried parsley flakes, dillweed, salt, garlic powder and celery seed and chill several hours to blend flavors. A delicious dip that's great for parties combines a pint of sour cream, a package of onion soup mix and four ounces of crumbled blue cheese, well mixed and chilled. These dips work well with crisp crackers and flatbreads, too.

2. Peanut power. A good high-energy treat that's even tasty for breakfast is a peanut butter and fruit sandwich. Spread two tablespoons of peanut butter and two tablespoons of ricotta cheese on whole-wheat toast. Sprinkle with cinnamon; top with a spoonful of honey and apple slices. Peanut butter also combines beautifully with mashed bananas on raisin bread; or with crisp, lean bacon slices on whole-wheat toast.

3. Gorp. This favorite snack of skiers and backpackers is a high source of energy and nutrition. Make up a big batch while you're at it—it keeps well in a screw-top glass jar. To make gorp, combine crunchy granola, raisins and dried fruits (snipped with wet scissors into small morsels), add unsalted nuts and mix well.

4. Peasant picnic. For centuries, European workingmen have enjoyed a simple, one-course meal of cheese and sausage or cured meat, sliced and tucked into split French or Italian bread. Here's how: Cut the bread into six-inch lengths, split lengthwise and fill with any cheese-meat combination that appeals. Try some of the tasty imported cheeses, such as Jarlsberg, Muenster, Gouda or Gruyère paired with liver sausage, Polish sausage, hard salami or pepperoni as an interesting change from processed cheese and bologna. Add crunchy pickles, mustard, fresh fruit and a beverage, and you have an unusual, nutritious meal.

Now, before we turn to overweight and underweight, a word about water. Yes, good old *aqua pura.* Water is essential to a well-balanced diet. If you don't drink enough, your body will not have enough fluid to absorb vitamins and minerals properly. Dr. Leroy Perry, who works with athletes, has developed a formula to figure the minimum amount of water you need, based on your body weight. The active teen-ager should figure one-half his or her body weight to equal the ounces of water needed daily. So a 120-pound girl would drink 60 ounces of water, or about seven 8-ounce glasses of water every day. (This includes water drunk in other beverages.) Less active people require water equaling one-third of their body weight; professional and Olympic-level athletes need a water intake equaling two-thirds of their body weight.

We should point out here that whenever you have special nutritional needs or problems, always ask your doctor. Only a doctor should decide whether you need a special diet, food supplements or vitamin prescriptions to improve or maintain your health. Earlier, we mentioned the danger of vitamin and diet fads. We want to reemphasize the point that you should not try diet drugs, "miracle" foods or crash diets that promise rapid results. If you are overweight or underweight, do ask your doctor's advice about a sensible diet program.

Both overweight and underweight are related to caloric intake. A calorie is simply a unit used to measure food energy. When food energy is consumed by the body but not used up by the body, it accumulates, adding body fat and weight. When not enough food energy is supplied to the body, underweight results.

Overweight is a particular problem among young adults. Overeating, disregard of sound nutrition, lack of exercise and emotional tension are four of the basic causes. It has been estimated that there are about 10 million overweight teen-agers in America today!

One pound of body fat contains 3,500 calories. So if you want to lose a pound a week, you would cut out 500 calories a day to achieve a seven-day total reduction of 3,500 calories. If yours is a well-balanced diet to begin with, then you merely *reduce the size of the portions you eat by about 25 percent.* Maintain a regular daily routine of exercise and sufficient sleep, and your body will achieve the proper balance of food intake to body use.

At the opposite end of the scale is the string bean. If you are underweight, you need to supplement your daily intake of foods with more high-calorie foods. But please keep in mind that the high-calorie foods you eat also should be rich in proteins, minerals and vitamins for healthy muscles and tissues. There are several ways to build up weight: daily outdoor exercise to tune up your appetite, using the scientific snacking principle, adding extras to your regular meals—such as an extra pat of butter on vegetables, mayonnaise on salads, milkshakes, ice cream and other healthful high-calorie foods. Don't try to gain weight all at once. Just as the fatties do, you should work toward a desired weight goal at a rate of a pound or so per week.

We titled this chapter "Food for Thought." Nutrition and weight control go hand in hand with exercise in achieving good looks and maintaining a high level of health and energy. So, do think about it. *Bon appetit!*

CHAPTER SEVENTEEN
FACING REALITY: DRUGS AND ALCOHOL

> Drugs offer an illusory security from
> adolescent anxieties, but the young people
> who seek security from drugs actually
> disrupt the process. They have chosen drugs
> instead of growing up. If they persist in that
> choice, they will not grow up.
> —*Dr. Mitchell S. Rosenthal*
> *President, Phoenix House*

Each and every one of us knows at least one person who is dependent upon drugs, alcohol or (the most dangerous) a combination of both. It is a bad enough problem when it occurs to older people, but it is tragic when it happens to teen-agers. We know that there is a 50-50 chance that a young person will have tried one or more mood-altering drugs by college age, and that 20 percent of all college-age people are fairly regular drug users. We also know that 70 percent of today's teen-agers do drink—including 62 percent of all seventh-graders. So it is nonsense to pretend that drug taking and drinking aren't a fact of life. It also is foolish for adults to say, "Stop! It's wrong, illegal, and will wreck your life" when they *themselves* have the same problems as teen-agers do.

So, what we are attempting in this new chapter is to present the facts as clearly as we can, about the *physical* realities involved. A lot of this material isn't generally known to the public, because it is gathered from medical journals and case histories, as well as from drug treatment experts and our own patient files. So we ask that you really take the time to sit down with this "heavy" stuff and study it. (And share it with your parents. They will learn something, too.)

First, let's consider *psychoactive,* or mood-altering drugs. This group includes marijuana, "angel dust" (PCP), LSD, amphetamines, tranquilizers and sleeping pills. Some of these chemicals, when they were first introduced, were hailed as a wonderful way to solve a wide range of human problems. First developed as a way to manage (not cure) psychotic patients, they became widely used by the general public—the cramming student, the tense businessman, the exhausted housewife. Last year, about 230 million prescriptions were written for these pills, enough to keep every man, woman and child in this country "up," "down," and "out of it" for a solid month!

Two of these drugs require in-depth discussion. The first is *marijuana,* the most commonly used drug. It is also the most controversial. Marijuana has been around a long, long time. The Chinese used it as early as 200 B.C. as a pain reliever and anesthetic. Later in India it was used for both medicinal and religious purposes. Priests took it to expand their minds to "reach God." It was introduced into the Western world in the middle of the nineteenth century by Napoleon's soldiers returning from war in Egypt. In America it was used to treat all sorts of ailments, including migraine headaches, before it was declared illegal.

In 1961, at the request of its Asian and African members, the United Nations recommended that worldwide cultivation of the marijuana plant be eliminated over the following twenty-five years. The Asians and Africans said that the widespread use of marijuana on their continents was associated with physical and mental disease as well as with "social stagnation." President Lyndon Johnson signed the so-called United Nations Single Convention in 1967.

It was at that very same time that millions of young Americans were beginning to smoke marijuana and enjoying its effect of "turning on." "Legalize pot!" became a campus war cry, supported by many prominent doctors and psychiatrists, who said that marijuana was not harmful or addictive. Well, more than a decade has passed since then, and during that time enough clinical evidence has piled up to indicate that marijuana does in fact have *serious physical effect upon the body,* as well as upon the mind. These effects are:

1. It remains in the body. Its active ingredient, *tetrahydrocannabinol* (THC), is deposited in the fatty outer membrane of body cells and stays there. One cigarette a week could cause a chronic effect. Says Dr. Hardin B. Jones, senior scientist at the Donner Laboratory of Medical Research, University of California: "With repeated exposure, THC accumulates in the body. The marijuana user is under the influence of the drug even between 'highs.' "

2. The THC in marijuana injures the brain-cell membranes. Says Dr. Jones, "When the fine, hairlike extensions of the brain cells that communicate with other brain cells are damaged, it is critical, for they are the mechanisms of the mind. It takes decades for irreversible brain changes to appear in the heavy drinker. In the marijuana smoker, irreversible brain changes may appear within three years." (The word *irreversible* means here that the brain cannot be returned to its normal state.)

3. Marijuana smoke, like tobacco smoke, may irritate the bronchial tubes. In milder form, this results in cough and sore throat. Studies by the President's Committee on Drug Abuse, Washington, D.C., indicate that excessive marijuana smoking, at the rate of 5 cigarettes a day over a three-month period, may cause emphysema, a serious lung disease.

4. THC in marijuana causes genetic malformation in the fetus in pregnant women. Its sedative effect leads to a lessening of the sexual drive after habitual use over a period of time.

5. It affects the body's red and white blood cells, causing a decrease in the amount of oxygen in the blood. Its use, therefore, is especially dangerous for those with heart disease.

6. Marijuana impairs visual perception and muscle control. Studies of the influence on drivers have shown that it reduces the driver's ability to judge distance, speed and road conditions.

7. It affects the stomach and intestines by diminishing the level of acid normally found in the stomach. When the acid level is lowered, ingested bacteria, which would be killed by the acid, survive and multiply in the body.

8. It produces hair and skin problems which are often severe. In our own practice we have seen more than 100 cases of excessive hair loss among both young men and women. We believe this skin and hair damage is related to the general cell injury caused by THC.

Those are the *physical* realities of marijuana. Now let us dwell briefly on the mood-altering and mind-bending dangers of this drug when used by your age group. Writing in the *Journal of the American Medical Association,* Dr. Harold Kolansky and Dr. William T. Moore of the Child Analysis Division, Philadelphia Association for Psychoanalysis, reported, "Thirty-eight individuals from age thirteen to twenty-four were studied over a period of five years. All showed adverse psychological effects. Of the twenty males and eighteen females, there were eight with psychoses; four of these attempted suicide."

Marijuana, in affecting the brain, at first stimulates the "pleasure centers" of the brain, making the user feel "high," have "creative thoughts" and so forth. After a number of years, as the THC is increasingly stored in the cells, ability to think logically is decreased and judgment, memory and logic are affected. During the teen-age years when your physical, emotional and mental processes are undergoing the most rapid change and development you will ever experience, excessive use of marijuana interrupts these normal processes. So, the President's Committee concludes that you can reach adulthood in years without achieving normal, adult mental functioning or emotional responsiveness if your system is loaded with THC through excessive use of marijuana.

Now for a few case histories:

John, a young graduate student, was typical of many patients who used marijuana every day. He could not sleep at regular hours and had trouble concentrating. In speaking he used all the current clichés and was unable to focus his attention. He came to see us regularly to argue about pot, and after a year he gave it up. But the effects of smoking so much marijuana over so long a period remained. Even today, John has to focus his attention consciously before he can think and act as other people do spontaneously. (Dr. David H. Powelson, Former Chief of Psychiatry, Cowell Hospital, University of California, Berkeley), in *Executive Health*

An eighteen-year-old boy who had smoked marijuana regularly for a three-year period became progressively withdrawn and depressed. His interest in astrology and Eastern religions increased. He became a vegetarian and practiced yoga. He had the delusion that he was a guru and eventually believed that he was the son of God who was placed on earth to save all people. Persuasion could not convince this young man to give up the drug, although he admitted that his symptoms resulted from drug use. After consultation he moved to the West Coast and continued his unproductive, aimless life, supported financially by his parents. (Drs. Kolansky and Moore), *Journal of the American Medical Association*

A sixteen-year-old girl who had no prior psychiatric difficulties smoked marijuana at first occasionally, and then three to four times weekly for a period of two years. She began to lose interest in academic work and became preoccupied with political issues. From a quiet and socially popular girl, she became hostile to her teachers and peers. She dropped out of school in her senior year of high school, which led to psychiatric referral. She refused to give up smoking marijuana and eventually became so depressed that she attempted suicide by hanging. After withdrawal from the drug, her depression and paranoid ideas slowly disappeared. Ten months of follow-up showed continued impairment of memory and thought disorder, marked by her complaint that she could not concentrate on her studies and could not transform her thoughts into written or spoken words as she had once been able to do. (Drs. Kolansky and Moore), *Journal of the American Medical Association*

Recently, a young girl visited our office, frantic about her severe loss of hair and excessive dandruff. Her appearance and her clothing were messy. A school dropout, she was living in a communal "pad" in New York's East Village. When we questioned her carefully, we found she was a constant user of pot. What could be done to save her hair? she begged. We told her to stop taking marijuana immediately, instructed her on proper scalp hygiene, prescribed a biological scalp lotion, an antiseborrheic shampoo and vitamins taken internally. Eight weeks later, her hair loss had been arrested and it was beginning to regain its sheen and thickness. She told us she intended to return home, to her parents and to school. (Dr. Irwin I. Lubowe)

To sum up, we find the observations of Dr. Powelson, who saw marijuana first take root on the Berkeley campus, especially important. He says that by the spring of 1970 he had studied hundreds of marijuana-using students and became convinced that his original opinion about the harmlessness of pot was wrong. He now believes that marijuana is the most dangerous drug we must contend with. Why?

1. Its early use is sneaky. Because the user feels "great," he cannot sense the mental and physical damage that is occurring.
2. Its continued use leads to delusional thinking. After one to three years of use the thought processes become abnormal.
3. There is a strong need to influence others into using the drug.
4. Marijuana users usually progress to more frequent use or to more potent varieties of pot. And they often progress to other, even more dangerous drugs. Most hard-drug users began on marijuana.
5. There is danger to those whose lives the pot smoker affects. Because marijuana accumulates in the brain, people who use marijuana are clinically "stoned" all the time. "Thus, we have reason to be concerned about public safety if airplane pilots,

firemen, policemen, surgeons and nurses are users of the drug," says Dr. Powelson.

The second psychoactive drug we want to tell you about in detail is PCP, or angel dust, the most lethal new drug around. What's more, its use is concentrated among teen-agers. The National Institute on Drug Abuse estimates that between 6 million and 7 million young people between the ages of twelve and twenty-five are using PCP today. Angel dust is PCP's most common name, but it also is known as "superjoint," "busy bee," "crystal," "peace pills," "green tea leaves," "elephant," and "cyclone." Most often it is sprinkled on marijuana, mint leaves or parsley and smoked. However, it also is snorted, taken by mouth or by intravenous injection.

As is true of so many of the chemical compounds that were first manufactured for medical *use* and not *abuse,* PCP, or phencyclidine, was developed as an anesthetic in the early 1960s for use on human beings. Early clinical studies quickly revealed it produced severe psychotic side effects and it was withdrawn for use on human beings. (Its only legal use today is as an anesthetic for monkeys and elephants, who do not suffer its side effects.)

The federal Drug Enforcement Administration has moved to curb illegal use of the drug (only five kilograms can be legally made each year for veterinary use) by placing it on its list of controlled compounds (along with other widely abused drugs) and monitoring its legal manufacture.

But the problem is, of course, that PCP is obtainable "on the street." Available in liquid, powder, tablet or rock crystal forms, it can produce tragic consequences for young people. Says David Hoover of the Drug Enforcement Administration, "Hallucinations and violent or aggressive behavior are only the mild effects of the drug. In some cases the drug can induce comas lasting a few hours to several weeks, or cause psychosis that closely resembles paranoid schizophrenia. *One* dose is enough to affect the user."

Frightening? We mean it to be. While by now most everyone has gotten wise to the dangers of LSD, its place is rapidly being filled by cheap, available PCP as a people destroyer. Here are its effects:

1. PCP is retained in the fatty parts of the brain cells, just like marijuana's THC—and LSD. A series of medical studies reported in *Clinical Toxicology* concluded that in human beings, this storage of PCP in the brain causes flashbacks (a "bad trip" is repeated in the mind over and over again) and mental symptoms resembling schizophrenia. This chemical damage also produces hallucinations, changes in body image (the user feels his arms are dead, or his legs are floating away), violent and murderous behavior, paranoia, stupor and coma. It often requires psychiatric hospitalization.

2. PCP affects the heart and lungs, causing increased heartbeat and high blood pressure. In some cases, death can result from respiratory failure.

3. PCP also causes loss of muscle coordination and numbness of the limbs, sweating, flushing, blurred speech and vision, dizziness and unpleasant nausea.

4. Finally, a report in the *Journal of the American Medical Association* states that in some cases people using PCP may suffer a "fatal hypertensive crisis" that will blow not just their minds, but their entire life-sustaining system.

Those effects are just the tip of the iceberg. It will take years more of intensive study to determine its long-range effects upon the body and brain. Its short-term effects are bad enough. Yet nearly one-third of young people reporting to drug treatment centers have tried PCP and about 20 percent use it regularly. At New York's Phoenix House, in just one month, seventeen out of twenty admissions to the group teen-age therapy program admitted to being PCP users. Says Phoenix House president Rosenthal, "Kids think that angel dust is not dangerous, that it's just a kind of super marijuana joint. The fact is, angel dust is so dangerous because it is unpredictable. It hits adolescents when they are more insecure, uncertain, frightened and more vulnerable than at any other time in their lives."

Here are summaries of three cases reported by Marcia Kramer in the *New York Daily News,* February 23, 1978:

> A teen-ager who was on an angel dust "high" stabbed his best friend four times. He said he had no recollection of the incident until his girl friend told him that his friend was in the hospital and it was his fault. He has now been in the Phoenix House program for four months without PCP.

> A young girl began smoking PCP three times a week when she was thirteen. Her parents did not know about her habit. Now seventeen, and a Phoenix House patient, she admits that while on the habit, she used to rob stores and gas stations, and then forget these incidents. Today, off PCP, she suffers from flashbacks, has a withdrawn, spaced-out manner and speaks in a whisper. Her caseworkers say this is probably due to her large continuing doses of angel dust over a four-year period.

> A pending criminal case describes a twenty-six-year-old man who shared a small apartment with his mother on New York City's Upper West Side. He smoked four joints of PCP and went home. There his mother was attacked with a knife and killed. His own hand was injured, but the next day he said that he had no recollection of the murder. On the living room wall, written in red marking pencil, were the words "I love my mother and didn't mean to kill her."

Some other "angel dust" incidents reported in *Time* magazine included a man in California who walked into a house at random, killed a baby and stabbed a pregnant woman in the stomach. Another Californian tore out both his eyes with his bare hands. Another bit off the breast of his girl friend.

Writing in *Woman's Day,* David Black described an ex-PCP user in his early twenties whom he interviewed as "a wizened old man. When he talks he blinks as though he has been startled awake. He chain-smokes cigarettes, punctuating his sentences with frequent coughs which sound like the rattling of seeds in a dried-out gourd."

So please, friends, steer clear. Don't be talked into trying

PCP by so-called "buddies" and don't be attracted by *head shops* that sell do-it-yourself drug equipment, ingredients and "turn-ons." These head shops, often masquerading as candy stores and often located near schools, sell all sorts of inhalants, herbal mixtures, cigarette papers and smoking implements.

While we don't have to dwell on the hard stuff—their dangers have been spelled out for a good many years and most teen-agers have become smart enough to avoid LSD, cocaine and heroin—we think it is important to review the prescription drugs. These are the tranquilizers, sedatives and stimulants, the "uppers" and "downers" that are as popular with parents as they are with their teen-age children. These, too, are psychoactive, or mood-altering drugs, and they can produce many of the physical and mental effects we've already described. They also are addictive.

Tranquilizers are the most widely prescribed class of drugs, used mostly to reduce feelings of anxiety. They also are prescribed for muscle relaxation. Some of the brand names are Valium, Librium, Miltown and Equanil. When their habitual use is stopped, the withdrawal symptoms can be painful and, in some cases, acute.

Sedatives are barbiturates that work to depress certain brain functions and induce a drowsy calm when used in small doses. In larger doses, the brain is depressed still further, causing sleep. Overdoses can depress the brain functions enough to cause coma and death. Some sedatives are Amytal, Seconal and Nembutal. Nonbarbiturate sedatives include Placidyl and Quaalude.

Stimulants are the opposite of sedatives. They work to briefly speed up mental functions to produce a wide-awake feeling. Amphetamines, such as Dexedrine, were also once widely used to encourage weight loss, but are now rarely prescribed because they have been found to be too addictive.

To avoid the pitfalls of the drug scene is difficult. Your success really depends upon your own sense of self-worth, as well as the good sense and understanding of your parents.

What happens when a teen-ager becomes addicted? Drug

treatment, as you know, is difficult, often expensive and not always successful. There are four basic ways of dealing with drug addiction in America today:

1. Hospitalization and/or imprisonment
2. Methadone maintenance, which is the substitution of methadone, a synthetic drug, for the user's drug, creating a new drug dependence
3. Psychotherapy, which is often lengthy, extensive and expensive, as well as uncertain in its results
4. Rehabilitation in a therapeutic community with other addicts.

Many experts feel that this last, close-knit community approach is the most successful and least costly method by far. Phoenix House, in New York City, and similar establishments such as Marathon House, DayTop Village, Odyssey and others throughout the country appear to be producing good results. At Phoenix House and similar community units, the live-in patients eat, work, study, fight and share in a drug-free atmosphere. Most importantly, as a Phoenix House staffer, an ex-addict, says, "We address ourselves to the real problem: growing up. Then the side effect, drug taking, goes away."

Facing reality about drugs includes *alcohol.* Alcohol is a drug. While it differs from the mood-altering drugs like THC and PCP in that it is not stored in the fatty brain tissues, it *does* affect the nervous system after reaching the brain. (Alcohol could also be called a food since it contains calories. But it is almost completely lacking in the nutrients needed for growth and good health.)

To research this section, we asked the aid of the National Clearinghouse on Alcohol Abuse, the National Institute of Alcohol Abuse and Alcoholism, the National Highway Traffic Safety Administration and others. As a result, we can scarcely see over the pile of clinical studies, articles, booklets, student surveys, scientific papers and computer printouts we have collected! But we are very grateful for their help, and have found some significant facts that come through loud and clear:

- Seventy percent of teen-agers drink. Some drink very occasionally, most drink regularly, a few heavily.
- Forty percent of you have tasted alcohol by the age of ten.
- Female teen-age drinking has increased sharply in the last twenty years, even though male teen-age drinkers still predominate.
- The typical teen-ager now drinks one to three times a week.
- Teen-agers with strong religious beliefs are more likely to abstain or drink sparingly than others.
- Less than half (42 percent) of you who drink do so at home with your parents.
- Teen-age drinking habits parallel those of their parents. Those whose parents drink are twice as likely to drink as those with nondrinking parents.
- Beer is the most popular alcoholic beverage among teen-agers, followed by wine, then hard liquor.
- Twenty-one percent of you have consumed five or more drinks in a typical drinking situation.
- Forty-five percent of you report having been drunk at least once in your life.
- Thirty-four percent of teen-age drinkers report that drinking is the cause of problems with school, parents, friends or the police.
- Almost 40 percent of all young people who drink, do so while sitting in a car or driving a car.
- Eight thousand teen-agers are killed each year in motor vehicle accidents where drinking is a factor. Forty thousand more are disfigured in these accidents.
- Sixty-nine percent of teen-age "problem drinkers" use one or more drugs. Marijuana-plus-alcohol is the most common combination.

What happens when you take a drink? It is quickly absorbed into the blood. Straight liquor is absorbed fastest. Drinks mixed with carbonated soda are next fastest, and those mixed with plain water are absorbed the most slowly. The liquor then passes directly through the walls of the stomach and the small intestine. Then the liver goes to work, oxidizing—burning up—some of the liquor. It takes the liver about an hour to burn up one highball, one glass of wine or one bottle of beer. Any remaining unoxidized alcohol remains in the bloodstream, where it then affects the brain.

In the brain, the alcohol slows down those portions of the brain that control judgment, thought and action. When these "controls" or inhibitions are slowed, the user feels relaxed, gay and carefree. This is why many people think of alcohol as a stimulant, or "upper." Actually, the opposite is true. Alcohol works to depress, not stimulate the nervous system. This depressant, or "downer" action increases as the user continues to drink. If enough alcohol is consumed, drowsiness, sleep or even, in extreme cases, death can result.

Alcohol also slows down the brain area that controls muscle coordination. So, it can interfere with movements of your arms and legs, speech and balance. It is the combination of lack of muscle control and decrease in judgment that makes the driving/drinking problem so crucial. We'll discuss that subject a bit later.

If you continue to drink alcohol faster than your body can burn it up, the alcohol concentration in the blood increases, the depressant action in the brain increases, you progressively feel more relaxed, less coordinated, then drunk, and finally—completely passed out.

Physical reaction to alcohol varies tremendously. Different people react differently to the same amount of alcohol. These reactions depend upon many different factors. For instance:

1. How fast do you drink? If you sip a drink containing half an ounce of pure alcohol slowly enough to last for a full hour, your body will burn up the alcohol at the same rate at which the bloodstream is absorbing it. If you gulp that same drink, you will quickly feel the effect and it will take about an hour for that feeling to wear off.

2. Have you eaten? If you have food in your stomach before drinking, that food slows down the rate at which the alcohol is absorbed into the bloodstream. Alcohol will then reach the brain at a slower rate than if you drink on an empty stomach. (Eating while drinking has the same beneficial effect, but to a lesser degree.)

3. What type of liquor are you drinking? Beer or wine has a slower effect than the same amount of alcohol consumed in the form of hard liquor. They also contain substances which slow down the absorption of the alcohol, resulting in lower alcohol concentration in the blood.

4. What are your weight and body chemistry? A small, thin person has less blood and other fluids in his body than a larger person. So the same amount of alcohol will be more diluted in a heavier person's bloodstream and will not affect him as soon or as strongly as it will the smaller drinker. Body chemistry is different in everyone. Some people can drink alcohol in quantity and appear to remain quite sober. Others react with nausea to even a tiny amount of alcohol.

Other factors are emotional: your mood, the social situation or setting, your attitude (and that of others) toward drinking.

The law is also involved in teen-age drinking. In most states, the "legal drinking age" refers to the sale or serving of alcohol in a public place. Usually this does not apply to drinking in a private home or nonpublic place. Some states do, however, forbid serving alcohol in homes to people under twenty-one. A few states permit the sale of alcoholic beverages to anyone over eighteen. Be aware of the liquor laws in your area and do not violate them.

One hundred million Americans drink today. Ninety percent of them, including teen-agers who drink, can handle their drinking behavior. The question of drinking or not drinking is purely a personal matter. It also can be a difficult decision, since your attitudes tend to be formed by your family, your friends, your religious beliefs, your age and the customs of your community. And whether you choose to drink or to say "No, thanks," you should feel comfortable with yourself about your reasons.

To help get things straight in your own head, try this self-quiz below. There are no right or wrong answers. The multiple choices are merely there to make you think (and to come up with better answers of your own). Try this quiz with your parents, and then again with your close friends. You'll find it leads to a fascinating "dialogue."

What Would I Do If . . .

My parents are nondrinkers. Do I
( ) make up my own mind about whether I will drink
( ) ask my parents' permission to drink
( ) accept my parents' attitude as my own, and not drink

I am permitted to drink at home. Do I
( ) assume I can drink elsewhere when I want to
( ) ask my parents for ground rules when drinking outside the home
( ) expect my parents to set up standards about drinking

I want to serve liquor at a party at my home. Do I
( ) make my own decision about what to serve
( ) ask my parents' okay
( ) make sure my friends' parents know and approve of my serving liquor

My date is drinking too much at a party. Do I
( ) ask my date to stop drinking
( ) suggest we both leave the party and return home immediately
( ) seek the help of a sober friend or parent

I am the only nondrinker in a group who urge me to drink. Do I
( ) take one drink, sip slowly and eat a lot
( ) ask for a nonalcoholic beverage instead
( ) refuse, with an excuse that may or may not be true

I feel myself getting high. Do I
( ) put down the drink and accept no more drinks
( ) ask someone to take me home
( ) lie down in another room

DRINKING PROBLEMS

There are special problems involved with drinking that do not necessarily involve the "problem drinker." There are two that have importance for teen-agers in particular.

1. Drinking and driving. We've already noted that about 40 percent of teen-age drinking takes place in cars. But did you know that traffic fatalities are the leading cause of death among teen-agers? Further, drivers under the age of eighteen already have the worst collision involvement of any age group when they have had nothing to drink. After just two or three beers, the teen-ager collision chances are *tripled*. So please study the accompanying table. It shows the effect of a number of drinks on responsible driving.

Wt.	Drinks Two-Hour Period 1½ ozs. 86° Liquor or 12 ozs. Beer											
100	1	2	3	4	5	6	7	8	9	10	11	12
120	1	2	3	4	5	6	7	8	9	10	11	12
140	1	2	3	4	5	6	7	8	9	10	11	12
160	1	2	3	4	5	6	7	8	9	10	11	12
180	1	2	3	4	5	6	7	8	9	10	11	12
200	1	2	3	4	5	6	7	8	9	10	11	12
220	1	2	3	4	5	6	7	8	9	10	11	12
240	1	2	3	4	5	6	7	8	9	10	11	12

Be Careful	Driving Impaired	Do Not Drive
BAC to .05	.05—.09	.10 & Up

This table shows the appropriate blood alcohol percentages after a number of drinks from one to ten. The left column of the table shows that depending upon your weight, one or two drinks rarely affect responsible driving. Beyond that, the probability of being seriously affected becomes much greater. *(Courtesy National Highway Transportation Safety Administration)*

The next important step is to establish a good, clear channel of communication with your parents about drinking and driving. Parents have not only a moral responsibility but a legal responsibility to protect the life and health of their children *and others* who may be involved in a driving accident. So we suggest you set up ground rules on such subjects as whether you are permitted to drive a car for a friend who has had too much to drink; whether you can stay over at a friend's house if you have had too much to drink; whether your parents will come and get you at any hour and any place under the same circumstance; whether they will pay for a taxi to get you home if your date is the drinker but incapable of driving safely.

If you are serving liquor at a party at your home, discuss in advance such rules as serving food with alcohol, not mixing drinks too strong, closing the bar at least one hour before your guests depart and refusing to serve another drink to a guest who has had too many.

2. Alcohol and other drugs. We think you've got the picture that drugs are dangerous enough all by themselves. The problem becomes even more serious when alcohol is added to the already explosive mixture in your brain. And as we have noted, problem drinking and marijuana use are highly related; 69 percent of teen-age problem drinkers use one or more drugs.

What many people don't realize, however, is that drinking combined with many legally prescribed drugs and nonprescription medicines can produce danger as well. In fact, the whole subject of what is termed "dual addiction" has suddenly surfaced as a major health problem among people of all ages. In many cases, the sufferer was completely unaware of the addiction problem. The National Institute on Drug Abuse estimates that in the year 1977, some 47,700 persons were admitted to emergency rooms from the effects of mixing alcohol and drugs. What are the "innocent" combinations to beware of? Don't mix alcohol with antibiotics, antihistamines, aspirin, sedatives, tranquilizers, high blood pressure medications, oral anticoagulants, oral antidiabetic preparations or nonnarcotic pain-killers!

PROBLEM DRINKERS

Drinking problems can happen to anyone—even the non-drinker who just happens to be a passenger in the wrong automobile! But problem drinkers are another kettle of fish. Among the 10 million Americans who are problem drinkers, it is estimated that 1.1 million are teen-agers. The dangers of drinking have been spelled out in this chapter. Briefly, any *negative* consequence of drinking, such as trouble with parents, friends, schoolwork and/or police is a clear signal of problem drinking to "escape" the stresses and strains of life.

There is plenty of help around for the teen-ager who wants to manage a drinking problem. Some national programs have adapted services originally developed for alcoholic adults to the special needs of young people. Alcoholics Anonymous, for example, reports an increasing involvement by young people. Alateen is the youth component of Al-Anon—a fellowship for friends and relatives of alcoholics—and is a primary treatment resource. Drug treatment centers also treat alcohol dependency. Some communities have special teen-counseling centers that include alcohol problems. Many schools and colleges have similar counseling and treatment setups. Churches and religious organizations also provide help.

Facing reality is the first step in acknowledging, then solving any problem. We sincerely hope this chapter has helped you to face the realities involved in the use of drugs and alcohol, and to reach some strong and sensible conclusions. For in the long run, no matter how much help you receive from others, the actual *doing* is up to you!

CHAPTER EIGHTEEN
CONTRACEPTIVES: WHAT THEY ARE, HOW THEY WORK

> I trust my children when they know the truth about things. It's when they *don't* know that I worry.
>
> —*"The Waltons" TV series*

Today, everyone learns the facts about sex, but contraceptive methods are still a source of confusion to many teen-agers. This confusion is compounded by the parent-child relationship. Many mothers feel if they discuss pregnancy prevention methods with their daughters, they are giving them the green light to participate freely in premarital sex. Their daughters, on the other hand, may not wish parents to know about their sexual activities and so seek contraceptive advice elsewhere. This makes many girls feel guilty. Others go the opposite route and just "don't bother" with any precautions. Out of every hundred girls who choose this course, eighty-five will be pregnant at the end of one year.

Then the situation is complicated even further by the attitude of many young males. They don't bother using a male contraceptive, and so place the entire responsibility on the female partners and their faith in the Pill. And finally, there are those who really don't know, or are too embarrassed to find out, about methods of birth control.

The result is that today's teen-age girls are becoming pregnant at the staggering rate of more than one million a year. That's one million unwanted, unplanned pregnancies. And frankly, the often-heard response, "Oh, well, I'll get an abortion," is not the solution. In fact, more and more doctors are convinced that an abortion can have emotionally painful consequences for a young woman. Other aspects of increasing sexual activity at an earlier and earlier age include an alarming rise in venereal disease (VD) and an increase in cervical cancer in younger women.

The word *contraception* means prevention of pregnancy. Contraceptives are the objects and methods used to achieve pregnancy prevention, or birth control. Without making any moral judgments, here are the facts about contraceptives for our male and female readers.

MALE METHODS OF CONTRACEPTION

There are far fewer ways and means for men to control pregnancy than women. There is one, however, that is effective, widely available without a prescription, has no harmful side effects and usually prevents venereal disease. It is an inexpensive product that is considered 90 percent effective. When used in combination with a female product, vaginal foam, it is almost 100 percent effective. Most experts agree that it is the best first method of birth control for teen-agers. So we have put it first on our list.

1. The *condom,* also known as a rubber or prophylactic, is an extremely thin rubber sheath worn over the penis. It works by preventing the male sperm from entering the vagina. It prevents VD in two ways: If the boy has the disease, the germs cannot leave the rubber-covered penis to infect the girl. If she has VD, the germs in her vagina cannot get through the rubber to infect him.

Condoms can be bought at drugstores without a prescription, where they also are known by such trade names as Trojan, Sheik and Peacock. They can be purchased in plain latex rubber or in prelubricated rubber form. Some have "reservoir" tips—half an inch left empty at the bottom, permitting the male sperm to be harmlessly ejaculated. If unlubricated condoms are purchased, they can be lubricated with contraceptive cream or jelly. (Don't use Vaseline for this purpose, however. It is a petroleum product and causes the condom to deteriorate.) Lubricated condoms are slightly more expensive and the silicone type is not greasy. Special condoms, known as "skins," are actually made from animal membrane and are thinner and less noticeable when worn. They are more expensive than those made of latex.

The condom is used by unrolling it on the erect penis after the male is aroused, but before actual genital contact begins. To be effective, it must be in place before the penis enters the vagina. Upon completion of the sexual act, special care should be taken to withdraw the covered penis carefully. This prevents any sperm from "leaking" into the vagina. Each condom should be used only once.

Do you have to be eighteen to purchase a package of condoms? In most states, you don't. And in some places where eighteen is the rule, the legislation is being changed to lower the age requirement, or abolish it altogether. Condoms also can be obtained at Planned Parenthood and similar clinics.

2. Withdrawal, or "pulling out" or *coitus interruptus,* is the technique of removing the penis from the vagina before the sperm is ejaculated into the vagina. It requires good timing and control on the part of the male to prevent any leakage of sperm both *before* and *after* ejaculation. This method has the advantages of having no side effects and needing no purchase or preparation, but its effectiveness in preventing pregnancy is very low.

3. Sterilization is 100 percent effective in preventing pregnancy. The male operation is called a *vasectomy,* in which the vas deferens that transmit the sex sperm are tied and cut. The operation itself takes about twenty minutes and is a safe surgical procedure. Having a vasectomy does not interfere with enjoyment of sex, as the male still can have an erection and ejaculate during intercourse. However, this is a permanent birth control method which means that the male can never father a child. Therefore, it is recommended for the teen-age male only in rare medical circumstances.

FEMALE METHODS OF CONTRACEPTION

There are lots of products, procedures and techniques designed for feminine birth control. They all work on the principle of preventing the female egg from the ovary from being fertilized by the male sperm. Some are highly effective, others are not. First, let's consider three products that require a doctor's examination, counseling, and prescription.

1. The *Pill* is the most widely used contraceptive in the United States and Canada today. Some 10 million females find it very satisfactory. It is almost 100 percent effective when taken faithfully, and is considered very convenient, since it is simply swallowed by mouth. However, it has some known side effects and is not always recommended for every young woman. A doctor, before prescribing the Pill, will perform a pelvic examination and take a careful medical history. If the Pill is judged to be a safe

Contraceptive devices shown are (from left to right) IUDs; condoms in boxes, dispenser packets and with and without reservoir tips; vaginal foam and insertion tube; the Pill in several of its forms; the diaphragm and vaginal jelly; and at right rear, contraceptive cream. *(Planned Parenthood Photo)*

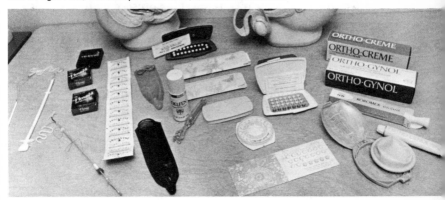

method for the individual girl, the doctor will prescribe one of the several Pill formulas available. Some formulas contain more hormones than others, and some are taken for twenty-one days every month, others for twenty-eight days.

What is the Pill? Basically it's a combination of progesterone and estrogen hormones, which chemically imitate pregnancy, causing the ovary to stop producing eggs. When this ovulation process is stopped, a woman cannot become pregnant, even when the male sperm enters her vagina. The Pill also works to prevent pregnancy by producing a thick mucus that prevents sex sperms from penetrating, and it also thins the lining of the uterus, making it difficult for any escaping egg to be nourished.

How is the Pill used? The twenty-one-day Pill is packaged in a compact with a pill for each of the twenty-one days. It is taken for fifteen days, starting five days after the beginning of the period. There is a rest for seven days, then the period starts again. Each cycle begins with a new compact. The twenty-eight-day Pill is taken every day of the month. During the menstrual period, the compact contains "blank" pills containing sugar or iron. You can see that in order to be effective, the Pill must be taken exactly as it is prescribed. One Pill swallowed on the evening of intercourse is useless. So is a Pill borrowed from a friend.

Is there an age limit? Girls over the age of eighteen can obtain them on their own request, as prescribed by a physician. Girls under eighteen must usually get their parents' consent, or be what is called an "emancipated minor"—one who is not financially supported by her parents. Further, if a girl is sexually active and wants contraceptive counseling, the Pill may be prescribed for her by a Planned Parenthood clinic.

As we said earlier, the Pill is not for everyone. There are side effects you should know about. Some of them are good, some are downright dangerous. In our medical practice, we also have seen that the Pill has a noticeable effect on the skin and hair.

Some of the benefits the Pill provides are correction of menstrual irregularity or excessive bleeding during the menstrual period. Others note a slightly increased bust size. We are also finding that the Pill can be helpful in the treatment of teen-age acne. It appears that the estrogen hormone in the Pill has the effect of reducing the flow of sebum, which contributes to skin eruptions. Therefore, we sometimes include the Pill as part of the total acne treatment for female patients. (This is not recommended for our male patients, though, since the hormone structure of the Pill could cause "feminine" sex characteristics to develop.) Other benefits of the Pill are the peace of mind it provides in sexual relationships by removing the tension and fear of unwanted pregnancy. And lastly, some previously infertile married women become joyfully pregnant after taking the Pill for some months, and then stopping.

So far, so good. But let's consider the possibly harmful side effects of the Pill, as well as those females who should not take it. Most of the side effects associated with the Pill are not dangerous, and many women experience little, if any of them. Some, however, may have nausea, vomiting, bleeding between menstrual periods, weight gain, breast tenderness or thinning hair. In rare cases, use of the Pill can cause blood clots, cerebral hemorrhage, liver tumors, high blood pressure, stroke or gallbladder disease. In some cases, when the Pill is taken during pregnancy, it has caused birth defects.

You shouldn't take the Pill (and your doctor shouldn't let you) if you smoke cigarettes. This is a major new warning issued by the federal Food and Drug Administration, and is based on their studies showing increased risk of heart attack and stroke for females who smoke while taking the Pill. These studies indicated that the risk increases with age and the amount of smoking, and if a woman has other conditions such as high blood pressure, overweight or diabetes, use of the Pill is dangerous indeed. And the doctor wouldn't dream of prescribing the Pill for those who are subject to those illnesses, or have cancer of the breast or sex organs, unexplained vaginal bleeding or are pregnant. Instead, there are alternate prescription methods of birth control that rate almost as highly as the Pill.

2. The *IUD,* or intrauterine device, is worn internally, and also must be prescribed and fitted by a physician. It is very effective in preventing pregnancy (more than 95 percent), has no chemical side effects and lasts as long as you wear it in the uterus.

IUDs resemble dainty pendants or earrings. Made of plastic or plastic wound with copper, they come in different shapes and sizes—loops, rings, coils and spirals, approximately one inch in length. Why and how they work so effectively is still a mystery! All we know is that they prevent the female egg from being fertilized or from becoming implanted in the uterus. They don't block the entrance to the womb or kill the male sperm, but somehow their shape and placement prevent pregnancy from occurring.

To fit an IUD, the doctor determines the size and shape most suited to the individual. The patient generally has a simple procedure performed in the doctor's office during her menstrual period. A local anesthetic is applied, and the IUD, which is very flexible, is straightened into a long, thin shape and placed inside an insertion tube. This tube, about the size of a soda straw, is gently pushed up through the vagina and cervix into the uterus. The doctor then expels the IUD from its tube, permitting it to curl and expand into its original shape. Most IUDs have threads attached, like those on tampons, permitting the wearer to check to see if the IUD is remaining properly in place.

Are there any side effects or drawbacks to the IUD? Some girls do experience cramping during the first few months the IUD is worn. Others find that the IUD is expelled during menstruation. (If this should occur, go back to the doctor and have it reinserted. *Never* try to pull out an IUD or put it in yourself.) The Food and Drug Administration also warns that the IUD may cause infection, bleeding and inflammation. If a female is prone to any pelvic infection or abnormality in the structure of the uterus, it will not be prescribed.

3. A third, very effective prescription contraceptive is the *diaphragm*. A traditional standby of female birth control, it is enjoying new popularity among many women because it has no side effects, such as those of the Pill or the IUD. Its pregnancy prevention rating is about 97 percent when it is used with a spermicidal cream or jelly.

The diaphragm is a soft rubber cone from two to four inches across, shaped like half an orange, with a flexible rim around the edge. Placed into the vagina before intercourse, it covers the cervix like a cup, protecting the uterus from the entry of the male sperm.

In prescribing a diaphragm, the doctor will first decide upon the right size. Then a teaspoon of spermicidal cream or jelly is placed in the center of the diaphragm and a bit rubbed around the rim. Then the edges are pressed together, the lips of the vagina are opened and the diaphragm is gently inserted into the vagina at an angle as far back as it will go.

This insertion technique must be practiced by the user until it becomes as automatic as the insertion of a tampon. Insertion must take place before intercourse. If the sexual act takes place more than two hours after insertion of the diaphragm, then, before intercourse, add more jelly or cream with an applicator, leaving the diaphragm in place.

After intercourse, the diaphragm must stay in place for six to eight hours to make sure that no active sperm remains in the vagina. Many doctors recommend applying additional jelly or cream with the applicator after intercourse as a *double check*.

The diaphragm is removed by hooking a finger under the rim, and gently pulling it out, bending it into the same shape as when inserted. After removal, it should be washed with soap and water and carefully dried. Before putting it away, sprinkle it with talcum powder to keep it soft and pliable. With care, a diaphragm can last over a year.

Lack of side effects and good protection against pregnancy are the benefits of the diaphragm when it is properly fitted by a doctor, the wearer is instructed in its use, and it is worn with vaginal cream or jelly applied *before* and *after* intercourse. Drawbacks of this method are that it must be placed within the vagina before intercourse, and some females find insertion a complicated process. However, we note that Planned Parenthood recently recommended more widespread use of the diaphragm because of its safety. Other statistics show that women who use the diaphragm have a lower rate of cervical cancer than those who use the Pill or the IUD.

Now let's turn to other methods of protection that don't require prescriptions, are available in drugstores and have no harmful side effects. While these "over-the-counter" preparations do not provide as high a percent of protection as the three prescription devices above, they can offer a fairly effective means of birth control when used properly.

4. Foams, creams and jellies are all products placed inside the vagina before and after intercourse. They contain a spermicidal agent that acts to kill the male sperm, and they help "block" the entrance of the sperm into the uterus. They are found in the "feminine hygiene" section of the drugstore, under a variety of trade names.

Vaginal foam is fairly effective when used alone—rating about 80 percent. When used by the female in combination with the male partner using a condom, it is, according to one expert, Dr. Gordon Jensen, "virtually 100 percent effective." The foam-condom combination, therefore, is especially recommended for youthful or occasional sexual partnerships.

Foam comes in a pressurized container with an applicator. The user inserts the foam-filled applicator high into the vagina, while lying on her back. It is important that the foam thoroughly coat and protect the cervix to stop the entrance of sperm. Foam must be applied before intercourse, and again after intercourse. Many doctors also recommend applying *double* the amount of foam suggested for added protection. Some well-known trade names for foam are Emko, Delfin Foam and Encare.

The vaginal creams and jellies found in the feminine hygiene section of the drugstore really aren't effective if they are to be the *only* birth control method used. They should be used only to coat the diaphragm as described earlier. Sold under such trade names as Delfin gel, Ortho-Gynol, Kormex and Lorphyn, they also can be used in combination with the condom worn by the male, but the effectiveness rating is lower than foam.

With all of these vaginal products, remember that they must be used before and after intercourse, a doubled application is more effective than a single one, and they must not be douched out afterwards.

5. The *rhythm method* is an ancient one. It is the only birth control method currently endorsed by the Catholic Church. Its rating is only about 45 percent as effective as the methods we've described above, so it cannot be considered dependable in preventing conception. It is a "natural" method, requiring no products or prescriptions, and has no side effects. Drawbacks are its lower degree of effectiveness in preventing pregnancy, the necessity of abstinence from sex during female ovulation, and the fairly complicated charting and temperature-taking, carefully carried out over a considerable period of time, that it involves. "Rhythm" refers to the female's own individual rhythm or cycle of her reproductive system. It means keeping a careful record or calendar of many monthly cycles to figure out an average of the most probable day for ovulation, or when the female eggs can be fertilized by the male sperm. Generally, ovulation occurs ten to fourteen days after menstruation, which means that the usual fertile time is midway between menstrual periods. Therefore, a safer time for sex would be just before, during or after the menstrual period itself. When ovulation occurs, the body temperature rises about five-tenths or six-tenths of a degree higher than normal body temperature. Therefore, some women use a basal thermometer to measure the body temperature every day, along with the chart. Once the time of ovulation is established, the female then does not have sex for at least eight days.

Of course, this method depends on very accurate charting and record-keeping over a long period in advance, and it is not at all successful for girls who have irregular periods, since the exact time of ovulation cannot be predicted accurately for each month.

6. *Sterilization* procedures are available that make the female incapable of bearing children. These are rarely done during the teen-age years. Briefly, there is tubal ligation, or "tying the tubes," an operation that usually is performed on an older woman at the time of delivery of her last wanted child. It involves tying off and cutting the Fallopian tubes, so that ova released from the ovary are absorbed into the body and do not become fertilized by sperm. A hysterectomy is another surgical operation that removes the entire uterus. This is performed for medical reasons other than preventing pregnancy, but it does have the same result. As with the male vasectomy, these operations do not interfere with the act of intercourse itself.

"NOTHING" METHODS

Even in our space-age world, myth and misinformation stubbornly persist. So, here's a rundown of some unreliable methods of birth control that do not work. One is the *douche,* which is a washing out of the vagina after intercourse. In addition to vinegar and water, soda pop and other home remedies, there are now all sorts of douches marketed with pretty names and fancy fragrances for "intimate feminine daintiness." Not only are they no good at preventing pregnancy, they can cause actual damage to the delicate tissues of the vagina, and can cause contact dermatitis and itching in the male partner as well as the female. Douches should only be used when prescribed by a doctor for a specific medical problem. Foaming tablets and suppositories, which are inserted into the vagina, do not prevent pregnancy. In fact most of them, such as Norforms, aren't intended for birth control use at all. And finally, hot baths, cold showers and such don't do a thing to kill the millions of sperm ejaculated during intercourse.

THE ALTERNATIVE METHOD

Finally, there is one completely 100 percent safe and effective birth control method that requires no prescriptions, devices, money or trouble. It has no harmful side effects, and is available everywhere.

We mean *abstinence,* or celibacy—having no sexual intercourse at all. You don't hear about this method as much as you do the others, but millions of young men and women practice it because they believe it is best for them at this stage of life.

Abstinence, according to one expert, Dr. Helen Kaplan, Clinical Associate Professor of Psychiatry at Cornell University Medical College, is a sign of maturity. "Sex should not be used as a competitive game," she says. "As people are maturing, not having sex is a constructive alternative. No sex is certainly better than destructive or neurotic sex. In fact, promiscuous sexual activity is more often a sign of compulsion rather than a sign of mental or emotional health."

Saying "yes" or "no" to sex is a difficult decision. It involves asking yourself some searching questions, and then giving yourself honest answers in return! Try these:

1. Do I want sex because it will make me feel more popular? Or mature?
2. Can I discuss sex and birth control openly with my parents and partner?
3. Do I ever use sex as a weapon to punish anyone else (partner, rivals, parents)?
4. Am I prepared to have a baby now? Or an abortion?
5. Is my current relationship with a partner based on affection, trust, and honesty?
6. Does early sex fit in with my personal beliefs and goals in life?
7. Can I handle it wisely?

These are questions that can only be answered by you. At least now, you have the facts upon which to base your own decisions. Good luck!

CHAPTER NINETEEN
WHAT'S THE PROBLEM?

In the first eighteen chapters of this book, we have discussed you, your body, your skin, your hair and the food you eat.

Now, we'd hate to think that you haven't read every single word (authors are funny that way), but in case you haven't, and as a handy guide, we've charted the basic problems discussed, along with their causes and treatment.

We hope you won't need to refer to it often!

THE PROBLEM	THE CAUSES
Acne	Hormonal imbalance causing overproduction of sebaceous glands; faulty diet and digestion; local infections; heredity; upset of the sympathetic nervous system; use of drugs; adolescence; use of the Pill
Alcohol, abuse of	Emotional, psychological and physiological factors; drinking too much, drinking in combination with drugs
Allergies	Foods; substances in the air (inhalants); substances that come into direct contact with the body; substances that enter the body (medications and insect bites)
Athlete's foot	Fungi and bacteria that breed on the skin, cause itching and blistering

THE TREATMENT	MORE ON THE MATTER
Consult your doctor for a program of medical treatment; keep skin, hair and scalp clean; shampoo and wash often; don't squeeze pimples; watch your diet; keep fit; stay away from drugs; try to stay on an even emotional keel	Refer to Chapter II: *Acne: The Teen-Age Problem;* Chapter XVI: *Food for Thought;* Chapter XVII, *Facing Reality: Drugs and Alcohol;* and Chapter XVIII, *Contraceptives: What They Are, How They Work*
This problem usually requires medical therapy as well as counseling; you'll find it covered in Chapter XVII	For a full discussion, see Chapter XVII: *Facing Reality: Drugs and Alcohol*
Determine, with your doctor, the cause of the allergy, which may be done through skin patch tests; follow the doctor's advice on preferred cosmetics, foods, clothing, etc., to prevent recurrence	Recheck Chapter IV: *Allergies, Itches and Infections;* also read Chapter VII: *Mostly for Misses* (cosmetic allergies); Chapter VIII: *Twenty to a Teen—Fingers and Toes* ("Rhoda's Red Hands"); and Chapter XII: *The Doctor on Dyeing*
Wash feet and soak in a medicated solution; keep toes aerated and separated; use antiseptic powder or lotion; change footwear frequently	See Chapter VIII: *Twenty to a Teen—Fingers and Toes* ("Andy's Athlete's Foot"); Chapter IV: *Allergies, Itches and Infections*

THE PROBLEM	THE CAUSES
Bad breath	Eating spicy, pungent foods; drinking; excessive smoking; tooth decay; mouth infection; infected tonsils; upset stomach
Baldness—alopecia	Radical changes in hormonal secretion combined with extreme emotional tension; excessive oiliness and dandruff; specific diseases and postpregnancy; disorders of adrenal and thyroid glands; drugs
Baldness—female pattern type	Unwise and overzealous use of hair preparations and rollers; some hairstyles; teasing; permanent wave preparations; hair straighteners; sprays, lacquers and bleaches

THE TREATMENT	MORE ON THE MATTER
Minor cases can be cured with a mouthwash rinse, mint tablet, etc.; for persistent cases, visit your dentist to determine whether it is a symptom of a more serious problem	Check Chapter VI: *Crisp and Clean*
See a dermatologist for treatment; many alopecia cases can be helped today through medication and diet	Read Chapter X: *Problem Hair: Too Little,* and Chapter XVII: *Facing Reality: Drugs and Alcohol*
Consult a dermatologist for treatment and hygiene routines; observe good health rules; follow sensible hair care procedures; ask your doctor about wiglets, wigs and hair switches to disguise a very serious condition	Study Chapter X: *Problem Hair: Too Little;* also read Chapter XII: *The Doctor on Dyeing* and Chapter XIII: *Coiffure Care*

THE PROBLEM	THE CAUSES
Baldness—male pattern type	Genetic or hereditary; increased excretion of androgen, the male hormone; metabolic disturbances; excessive dandruff; nutritional disorders; infections; scalp injury
Birth control, means of	Dangers of unwanted pregnancy, abortion, and serious emotional problems that can occur if teens are ignorant about contraceptives and their use
Birthmarks and scars	Spotty skin pigmentation; injury to the skin; also congenital
Blisters	Pressure and friction on a localized area of the skin; severe burn
Contraceptives—see *Birth control, means of*	

THE TREATMENT	MORE ON THE MATTER
Observe complete hair cleanliness routines and proper diet; consult a dermatologist to determine the specific cause of the condition (in some cases, a complete physical and laboratory studies may reveal a body disorder as the cause)	See Chapter X: *Problem Hair: Too Little* and Chapter XIV: *Mostly for Men*
Know the facts!	Study Chapter XVIII: *Contraceptives: What They Are, How They Work*
Conceal the birthmark or scar with a cosmetic cover-up preparation; a dermatologist also can treat a serious condition by freezing, planing and other surgical techniques	Read Chapter VII: *Mostly for Misses*
Prevent blisters by wearing properly fitted shoes, protective socks and gloves for sports; if infected, see a doctor for treatment	Review Chapter VIII: *Twenty to a Teen—Fingers and Toes* ("Barney's Blisters") and Chapter XV: *Fitness: Fun and Games*

THE PROBLEM	THE CAUSES
Corns and calluses	Pressure on skin due to too-tight or improperly fitted shoes
Dandruff	Faulty diet; emotional tension; hormonal disturbance; infection due to disease; injury to the scalp; unwise or excessive use of hair preparations; hereditary factors; drugs
Diet, faulty	Poor eating habits; junk foods; fad diets; overeating; undereating
Drugs	Emotional and psychological factors; lack of knowledge about their effects; pressure from others

THE TREATMENT	MORE ON THE MATTER
Soak in hot water; apply salicylic acid plaster; surround area with protective pad until corn or callus can be removed	Read Chapter VIII: *Twenty to a Teen—Fingers and Toes* ("Corns and Calluses") and Chapter XV: *Fitness: Fun and Games*
Make sure yours is a well-balanced diet; avoid butter, chocolate, nuts, shellfish, iodized salt and fried foods; keep hair and scalp clean; shampoo regularly; use hair preparations wisely; get plenty of fresh air and exercise; consult your doctor for treatment of severe case	See Chapter IX: *What's on Top?;* also read Chapter XIII: *Coiffure Care,* Chapter XIV: *Mostly for Men,* and Chapter XVII, *Facing Reality: Drugs and Alcohol*
Eat the right foods, choosing your daily nourishment from each of the five basic food groups	Review Chapter XVI: *Food for Thought*
Understanding drugs is the best preventive medicine; both the mind and the body must often be treated to stop the habit and its harmful side effects effectively	Study Chapter XVII, *Facing Reality: Drugs and Alcohol*

THE PROBLEM	THE CAUSES
Dry hair	Underproduction of the sebaceous glands; excessive permanent waving, bleaching, tinting, etc.; overexposure to drying effects of weather
Dry skin	Extremes of temperature; underproduction of the sebaceous glands; excessive use of irritating alkalies and harsh soaps; heredity
Facial scarring	Severe acne
Gonorrhea	A bacterium transmitted through sexual intercourse which affects the vagina and urethral area

THE TREATMENT	MORE ON THE MATTER
Use a dry hair formula shampoo, cream rinses, vegetable oil-based dressings and hair conditioning sprays; avoid overtreatment of hair and outdoor exposure	Check over Chapter IX: *What's on Top?;* Chapter XII: *The Doctor on Dyeing;* Chapter XIII: *Coiffure Care;* and Chapter XIV: *Mostly for Men*
Hydrate the skin with a balance of moisturizing creams and oils; cleanse gently; use cream formula cosmetics and lotions, moisturized shave creams; eat a well-balanced diet containing plenty of Vitamin A; protect skin from weather	Refer to Chapter III: *One Extreme to the Other;* Chapter V: *Suntan: Delight or Danger?;* Chapter VI: *Crisp and Clean;* Chapter VII: *Mostly for Misses;* and Chapter XV: *Fitness: Fun and Games*
Recommended ways of removing scars are dermabrasion, in which scar tissue is planed away; peeling, a chemical means of correcting shallow pits; and chemotherapy, for more serious cases; all three are medical procedures	Read Chapter II: *Acne: The Teen-Age Problem*
Prevention is the best treatment, through use of the male contraceptive (condom); medical treatment consists of antibiotic therapy	Review Chapter IV: *Allergies, Itches and Infections* and Chapter XVIII: *Contraceptives: What They Are, How They Work*

THE PROBLEM	THE CAUSES
Herpes	A highly infectious virus transmitted by the sexual act; type I affects the face, type II the genital area
Hirsutism and hypertrichosis	Glandular imbalance, such as abnormal functioning of pituitary or adrenal glands; malfunctioning of female ovary; heredity
Infections	Eczema; fungi; bacteria; venereal diseases; viruses, etc.
Ingrown toenails	Improper cutting of toenails and ill-fitting shoes that don't conform to the shape of the foot
Insect bites, allergy to	Toxic substances deposited into the skin by the bite or sting of a mosquito, bee, wasp, hornet, yellow jacket, flea, etc.

THE TREATMENT	MORE ON THE MATTER
There is *no* effective cure for herpes, other than the preventive use of contraceptives	Study Chapter IV: *Allergies, Itches and Infections* and Chapter XVIII: *Contraceptives: What They Are, How They Work*
Temporary removal of unwanted hair by plucking, shaving, abrasion, wax and chemical depilatories; also permanent removal by electrolysis	Read Chapter XI: *Problem Hair: Too Much;* pay special attention to the discussion on hair removal techniques
All serious infections need a doctor's immediate care	Check Chapter IV: *Allergies, Itches and Infections;* also see Chapter VIII: *Twenty to a Teen—Fingers and Toes*
Alter growth pattern of the nail by putting medicated cotton between nail and skin; apply antibiotic ointment and compress; if infection sets in, see your doctor for treatment	Review Chapter VIII: *Twenty to a Teen—Fingers and Toes* ("Ira's Ingrown Toenails")
Protect yourself with insect repellent; learn emergency techniques for dealing with severe bites or stings; obtain aid from your doctor to relieve painful symptoms or to desensitize your body to the bites or stings	Read over Chapter IV: *Allergies, Itches and Infections;* pay special attention to procedures for dealing with severe bites or stings

THE PROBLEM	THE CAUSES
Oily hair	Overproduction of the sebaceous glands; excessive dandruff; faulty diet; glandular imbalance
Oily skin	Overproduction of the sebaceous glands; faulty diet containing an excess of fatty and greasy foods; adolescence
Overbleached and tinted hair	Damage to hair and scalp due to dye and bleach chemicals; hair straighteners and stripping
Overweight	Overeating; disregard of sound nutrition; lack of exercise; emotional tension; glandular imbalance

THE TREATMENT	MORE ON THE MATTER
Shampoo hair twice a week with an antidandruff or castile soap shampoo; eat a well-balanced diet, staying away from greasy and fatty foods; keep hairstyle manageable and easy to care for	Check Chapter IX: *What's on Top?;* Chapter XIII: *Coiffure Care* and Chapter XIV: *Mostly for Men*
Keep face, neck and scalp scrupulously clean with a detergent or astringent cleanser; avoid greasy cosmetics and hair dressings; cut down on fatty and greasy foods	Refer to Chapter II: *Acne: The Teen-Age Problem;* Chapter III: *One Extreme to the Other;* Chapter VI: *Crisp and Clean* and Chapter VII: *Mostly for Misses*
Prevent damage through correct application of hair color, use of a precoloring sensitivity test; avoid overexposure of color-treated hair to the sun; use a neutral or special shampoo for color-treated hair; avoid drastic color changes, hair straighteners; in severe cases, consult a dermatologist for treatment	Study Chapter XII: *The Doctor on Dyeing* and Chapter XIII: *Coiffure Care*
Learn to eat wisely, choosing foods from the five basic food groups; limit calorie intake to help reduce weight; get plenty of daily exercise	Read Chapter XV: *Fitness: Fun and Games* and Chapter XVI: *Food for Thought*

THE PROBLEM	THE CAUSES
Perspiration	Heavy flow of fluid from eccrine and apocrine glands; emotional tension; strenuous physical exertion
Poor muscle tone and coordination	Lack of daily exercise; faulty diet; drugs; alcohol
Psychoactive Drugs	A group of chemicals that affect the nervous system, including marijuana, "Angel Dust," LSD, amphetamines, tranquilizers and sleeping pills.
Prematurely gray hair	Defect in hair pigment mechanism formation; often hereditary
Ringworm—see *Athlete's foot*	
Split nails	Heredity; deficient diet; in some cases may also be a symptom of a more serious disease

THE TREATMENT	MORE ON THE MATTER
Keep body clean with frequent bathing or showering; use a deodorant chemical between baths; keep clothing clean and well aired between wearings	Read Chapter VI: *Crisp and Clean*
Eat your daily ration of muscle-building foods; exercise every day; avoid drugs and alcohol	Check out Chapter XV: *Fitness: Fun and Games* and Chapter XVI: *Food for Thought;* Chapter XVII: *Facing Reality: Drugs and Alcohol,* explains the effects of both upon muscular coordination
Nothing medical can be done if hair has lost its color; however, hair can be rinsed, tinted or dyed if you wish	See Chapter IX: *What's on Top?* and Chapter XII: *The Doctor on Dyeing*
Eat a well-balanced diet; try unflavored gelatine as a protein additive to the diet; use a nail-hardening polish; if trouble persists, see your doctor	Read Chapter VIII: *Twenty to a Teen—Fingers and Toes* ("Sally's Split Nails")

THE PROBLEM	THE CAUSES
Sunburn	Overexposure to burning rays of the sun that in some cases produces dangerous effects such as skin cancer, melanoderma, polymorphous light eruption, chloasma, etc.
Syphilis	Spirochete bacterium which starts as a sore on the genitals and may spread to other areas of the body; is transmitted through sexual intercourse
Tooth decay	Food particles lodged in the mouth, which turn into acids that destroy tooth enamel and cause gum infection
Underweight	Lack of enough healthful high-calorie foods in diet; lack of well-balanced diet; emotional tension; lack of proper exercise and rest; drugs
Warts	A wart virus that causes regrowth of tissue; warts can be spread by contact or rubbing

Venereal disease (VD)—see
Gonorrhea; Herpes; Syphilis

THE TREATMENT	MORE ON THE MATTER
Limit tanning time; sunbathe in relation to weather and locale; use a chemical sunscreen to filter burning rays; protect skin and hair; treat a sunburn medically—if painful, consult your doctor	Check out Chapter V: *Suntan: Delight or Danger?*; also read Chapter VIII: *Twenty to a Teen—Fingers and Toes* ("Barney's Blisters") and Chapter XV: *Fitness: Fun and Games*
Prevention is the best treatment, through use of the male contraceptive (condom); medical treatment is by antibiotics	Read Chapter IV: *Allergies, Itches and Infections* and Chapter XVIII: *Contraceptives: What They Are, How They Work*
Brush teeth after eating; massage gums; avoid decay-building foods; visit your dentist regularly for cleaning and cavity checkups	Read Chapter VI: *Crisp and Clean*
Eat your full quota of foods each day from the five basic food groups; supplement your daily intake with healthful high-calorie foods; increase appetite by daily exercise; get plenty of sleep and rest	Check Chapter XV: *Fitness: Fun and Games* and Chapter XVI: *Food for Thought*
Warts will often disappear by themselves; if bothersome, such as plantar warts, they can be removed by a doctor, either chemically or by electrodesiccation	See Chapter VIII: *Twenty to a Teen—Fingers and Toes* ("Wally's Warts," "Plantar Warts")

GLOSSARY

ACID MANTLE   Protective secretion on the skin surface, acid in composition.

ACNE   A skin disorder caused by inflammatory changes of sebaceous glands, manifested by external blemishes.

ACTH   A hormone secreted by the pituitary gland and stimulating to the adrenal glands.

ADRENAL GLANDS   Pair of ductless glands situated above the kidneys.

ALBINISM   Absence of pigment in the skin, hair and iris of the eye.

ALCOHOL   A pure ethanol chemical which when imbibed causes alternate stimulation and depression that can be addictive. Its effects are extremely harmful and may produce permanent mental depression and injure the genes.

ALKALINE   Having the chemical properties of an alkali, or substance to neutralize acids.

ALLERGY   An abnormal or altered sensitivity in the body to a specific substance (allergen), resulting in a sensitivity to certain foods, pollen, flowers, cosmetics, etc.

ALOPECIA   Loss of hair from the scalp which may be due to hormonal or emotional causes, overzealous cosmetic processes, or termination of the use of the birth-control Pill.

ALOPECIA AREATA—spotty baldness.

ALOPECIA TOTALIS—baldness of the entire scalp.

ALOPECIA UNIVERSALIS—baldness of the entire body.

AMINO ACIDS   The end products of protein digestion; natural protein building blocks essential for life and cellular activity.

ANDROGEN   Male hormone secreted by adrenal glands.

ANGEL DUST (PCP)   A hallucinogenic agent which when inhaled may cause quite injurious effects on the nervous system.

ANHIDROSIS   Absence of perspiration.

ANTIBACTERIAL   Destructive to or preventing the growth of bacteria.

ANTIBIOTIC   A substance derived from a mold or bacterium that inhibits the growth of microorganisms (bacteria). Penicillin and mycin drugs are most frequently used antibiotics.

ANTIBODY   Any substance in the blood that kills or prevents the growth of disease organisms, or neutralizes their poisons.

ANTIHISTAMINE   Drug having an action specifically antagonistic to that of histamine. Used in the treatment of allergic symptoms such as itching or hay fever.

ANTIPERSPIRANT   A preparation, usually an aluminum compound, that reduces the flow of perspiration of the sweat glands.

ANTISEPTIC   A substance used to destroy bacteria or inhibit their growth.

APOCRINE GLAND   Sweat gland located in axilla, breasts or pubic area—has special odor.

BALDNESS (FEMALE PATTERN)   An acquired type of baldness seen in women. It is related to incautious use of hair cosmetics.

BALDNESS (MALE PATTERN)   Common baldness; a type of baldness that is usually inherited.

BENZOCAINE   Local anesthetic which is used in post-sunburn lotions.

BIRTH-CONTROL PILL   A pill which contains the hormones progesterone and estrogen and is taken for fifteen days after the conclusion of the menstrual period.

BIRTHMARK   A circumscribed growth on the skin evident at birth. It is also referred to as a nevus or angioma.

BLACKHEAD   A small plug of fatty matter (sebum) blocking the duct of a sebaceous gland. It is also called a comedo.

BLEACHING AGENT   In reference to hair, an agent, usually a peroxide, which reduces the dark melanin in the hair to a lighter shade.

BULLOUS   Pertaining to blister formation, as in tinea pedis.

BUROW'S SOLUTION   Soothing solution, containing aluminum acetate, used in compresses.

CALAMINE LOTION   Soothing medicated lotion, pink in color.

CALORIE   A heat unit. In common usage, it refers to the food value of a particular foodstuff.

CAPITIS   Pertaining to the head.

CARBOHYDRATE   Sugar or starch.

CHIGNON   A round or curly mass of artificial or natural hair.

CHLOASMA   Pigmented patches of irregular shape and size, usually occurring on the skin of the face. They are also called liver spots.

COMEDO, COMEDONES   See BLACKHEAD.

CONDOM   A rubber sheath which is applied over the penis during sexual intercourse to prevent pregnancy.

CONTRACEPTIVE   An agent used to prevent pregnancy.

CONTRACEPTIVE FOAM   A foaming mixture which is inserted in the vaginal tract to cover the opening of the cervix and thus help to prevent impregnation.

CORTISONE   Steroid produced by the adrenal cortex.

CRASH DIET   A diet which is followed over a short period of time and in which there is a marked decrease in the intake of calories below that needed for a normal metabolism. Harmful medical symptoms can result.

CROWN   The topmost part of the head.

CUTANEOUS   Pertaining to the skin.

CUTICLE   The epidermis, or very thin outer layer of the skin or hair.

CYST, SEBACEOUS   A rounded tumor of variable size due to retention of secretion in the sebaceous follicle.

DANDRUFF   Pityriasis, scurf or abnormal shedding of scalp. Also called seborrhea capitis.

DEPILATION   Removal of hair by chemical or mechanical means.

DEPILATORY   A substance used to dissolve or remove hair.

DEPRESSANT DRUGS   Barbiturates. Also called barbs and goof balls. Can be physically addicting.

DERMABRASION   Removal of external layers of the skin by means of a rotary brush.

DERMATITIS   Inflammation of the skin.

DERMATOSIS   A noninflammatory disease of the skin.

DETERGENT   A salt of fatty acid which reduces surface tension and causes foaming when applied to skin or scalp; used in cleansing, in a manner resembling soap, but differs from soap in other respects.

DHA   Dihydroxyacetone—a chemical which produces a nonprotective, artificial tanning of the skin.

DIAPHRAGM   A rubber protective shield which is placed over the opening of the cervix before sexual intercourse in order to prevent pregnancy.

DISINFECTANT   An agent used to diminish the growth of bacterial organisms.

DYE   Artificial organic chemical used to change the color of the hair. Too frequent use may be harmful.

ECCRINE GLAND   Small sweat gland with opening on surface of skin.

ELECTROLYSIS   Decomposition of body tissues by means of electricity. The term is particularly applied to the destruction of hairs by this means.

ENDOCRINE   Pertaining to glands which secrete hormones; i.e., the thyroid, adrenal and pituitary glands.

ENZYME   A complex organic substance which reflects the rate of chemical reactions.

EPIDERMIS   The outer layer of the skin.

EPILATION   Removal of superfluous hair from the skin.

ERYTHEMA   Superficial reddening of the skin caused by increased circulation.

ESTROGEN   A female hormone produced especially by the ovaries.

EXCORIATION   Act of stripping or tearing off the skin (may be due to a neurotic state).

FATS   Chemically, fats are esters of certain acids, such as oleic, stearic, or palmitic acid. Fat is one of the three most important sources of calories in food.

FOLLICLE   The depression in the skin containing the hair and the opening of the sebaceous gland.

FRECKLES   Irregular collections of melanin in the skin, accentuated by exposure to the sun.

FUNGICIDE   A chemical that destroys fungi upon topical application.

FUNGISTAT   A chemical that prevents the growth of fungi. For example, griseofulvin, when taken internally, acts as a fungistat, as do parahydroxybenzoates when applied externally.

FUNGUS   Colorless plant. Unable to make its own food (since it lacks chlorophyll), it lives on other living or dead organisms.

FURUNCLE   Infection of a hair follicle, which becomes reddened and painful; a boil.

FURUNCULOSIS   Generalized occurrence of boils.

HANGNAIL   Overgrowth of the cuticle at the base of the nail.

HEROIN   A narcotic agent which is introduced into the body and used illegally as a hallucinogenic agent. It is addictive and may cause serious harmful effects to the nervous system and the genes. Methadone is now being used in the treatment of heroin addiction.

HERPES I   Condition marked by formation of vesicles, or blisters, due to virus, in groups on face or lip. Popularly known as "fever blisters."

HERPES II   Shingles; vesicular (blisterlike) inflammation usually appearing along the course of the cutaneous nerves. May also affect the eye branch of the facial nerve.

HIRSUTISM   Abnormal or excessive hair growth on the body.

HIVES   A disease of the skin characterized by the development of wheals, or elevations of the skin, containing fluid. Usually due to an allergic reaction.

HORMONE   A biochemical substance that is produced by an endocrine gland and is secreted into the bloodstream to stimulate the activity of body function; for example, estrogen, androgen or thyroxin.

HYPERHIDROSIS   Excessive perspiration. Usually becomes visible, in contrast to so-called insensible perspiration, which is invisible.

HYPERKERATOSIS   Thickening of the external layer of the skin as observed in seborrheic keratosis.

HYPOALLERGENIC COSMETICS   Cosmetics which contain very little of any known skin allergen or irritant, for use by persons allergic to ordinary cosmetics.

IMMUNITY   Condition that exists when the body defenses are able to react successfully to a disease or allergen.

IMPETIGO   A contagious disease in which the primary lesion ruptures and becomes covered with a thick yellowish crust.

INDUSTRIAL DERMATOSIS   Dermatosis incident to the patient's occupation in industry.

INFECTION   The invasion of the body tissues by disease-causing agents such as bacteria, fungi or viruses.

INFECTIOUS HEPATITIS   Viral inflammation of the liver, with evidence of jaundice.

INFLAMMATION   The reaction of the body to irritation or infection, with accompanying redness, pain, heat and swelling.

INGUINAL   Relating to the groin.

INTERTRIGO   Chafing, inflammation of opposing surfaces of the skin, as in the groin.

IODINE   A nonmetallic element found in shellfish. Irritating in acne and seborrhea.

KERATIN   A proteinlike substance forming the chemical basis of epidermal tissues such as horn, hair, nails, feathers, etc.
KERATINIZATION   The process of development and growth of skin from the basal cell layer to the outermost layer.
KEROLYTIC   Agent for the removal of skin oil.

LANOLIN   Purified wool fat used as an emollient for the skin.
LESION   Wound, injury or change in the tissues; one of the individual points or patches of a skin disease.
LIVER SPOTS   See CHLOASMA.
LOTION   Liquid medication prescribed for soothing the skin.
LSD   D-lysergic acid diethylamide, a dangerous drug that can distort perception and affect the body adversely. Also called acid.

MACULE   Flat localized area, usually reddened, on the skin.
MALIGNANT   Cancerous; said of a change in the tissues that may spread.
MARIJUANA   Drug made from leaves, flowering tops, and resin of the Indian hemp plant. Also called pot, grass, weed, tea, Mary Jane.
MELANIN   Brownish pigment that gives the natural color to the skin; it is increased after sunburn.
MELANODERMA   Excessive pigmentation following an inflammation.
MILIARIA   A rash, most common in summer, due to collection of sweat in the closed openings of the sweat ducts; it is accompanied by itching and discomfort.
MITE   Itch parasite that causes scabies.
MOLE   A birthmark that is usually present at birth and may grow larger after adolescence.

OCCUPATIONAL DERMATITIS   Inflammation of the skin due to an irritant or allergen encountered in the course of one's work.
OINTMENT   A medicated, semisolid mixture used externally, usually containing petrolatum or lanolin, and active therapeutic agents.
-ONYCHIA (Suffix)   Pertaining to the nails.
ONYCHOMYCOSIS   Fungous infection of the nails.
OPHTHALMIC   Pertaining to the eye.
OXIDATION   Chemical union of oxygen with another substance.

PAPULE   Localized elevation of the skin that may vary in size; contains no fluid.

PARASITE INFECTION   Dermatitis caused by an external parasite, as in scabies or pediculosis.

PARONYCHIA   Infection of the skin margin or cuticle covering the proximal part of the nail.

PASTE (MEDICATED)   Semisolid, thick ointment, usually containing petrolatum.

PATCH TEST   A test used to identify allergens. A small amount of the possible offending material is applied to the skin for forty-eight hours to determine the sensitivity of the user. A patch test should be made before application of hair dye, hair bleach or eye shadow.

PEDICULOSIS   Infestation with lice.

PEDICULOSIS CAPITIS—The presence of lice in the hair of the head.

PEDICULOSIS CORPORIS—The presence of lice on the body.

PEDICULOSIS PUBIS—The presence of lice in pubic areas.

PCP   Phencyclidine, popularly called "angel dust," "superjoint," "crystal," etc.; a dangerous psychoactive drug, illegal for use on humans

PENICILLIN   An effective antibiotic discovered by Fleming; can be given orally or by hypodermic injection.

PERMANENT WAVE   Cosmetic treatment, using the chemical glycolic acid, which curls the hair.

PIGMENT   Coloring matter; in the skin or hair, melanin granules.

PILO-SEBACEOUS UNIT   A unit or system in the skin hair follicle containing hair and sebaceous gland.

PITYRIASIS CAPITIS   A scaly inflammation of the scalp marked by dry dandruff, usually accompanied by itching.

PLANTAR WART   Wart on the sole of the foot.

PLAQUENIL   Antimalarial drug used to treat lupus erythematosus and to protect the skin from the sun.

POLYMORPHOUS LIGHT ERUPTION   Sensitivity and rash of skin developing after exposure to sun.

PPD   Paraphenylene diamine, the aniline dye most popular for dyeing hair.

PROTEIN   A basic food substance, containing nitrogen, characteristic of all living matter. Found in meats, poultry, fish, dairy products, etc.

PUSTULE   A circumscribed collection of infectious material or pus resulting from infection of a papule.

PYODERMA   Pus-forming infection of the skin.

RADIATION THERAPY   X-ray treatment of superficial type used in treatment of skin diseases.

RHUS DERMATITIS   Dermatitis caused by poison ivy plant.

RINGWORM   Infection of the skin due to fungi. It is scientifically called *tinea*. Various types are *tinea capitis* (scalp); *tinea crura* (groin); *tinea pedis* (feet); *tinea corpora* (body); *tinea ungum* (nails).

SCALE   A thin layer of horny epidermis.

SCAR   Permanent damage to the deeper layers of the skin following surgery or wound.

SCRATCH TEST   Test made to determine the possibility of the subject's being allergic to the test substance.

SEBACEOUS GLAND   Oil gland of the skin which secretes sebum.

SEBORRHEA   Overactivity of the sebaceous glands.

SEBORRHEA CAPITIS   Seborrhea of the scalp, commonly known as dandruff; pityriasis.

SEBUM   The fatty or oily secretions of the sebaceous glands; serve to lubricate the skin.

SEROLOGY   Blood test to determine the presence of syphilis.

SEX HORMONES   Secretions of the internal glands that cause sexual maturity. The female sex hormones are known as estrogens; male sex hormones are androgens and testosterone.

SHINGLES   See HERPES II.

STIMULANT DRUGS   Benzedrine, dexedrine, and methedrine. Also known as pep pills, bennies, dexies, and speed. Can be physically addicting.

STRIPPING HAIR COLOR   Removal of one color and then introduction of another. Very damaging to hair.

SULFA DRUGS   Synthetic anti-infective drugs such as sulfadiazine, sulfapyridine and sulfathiazole, which are used in the treatment of skin and other diseases.

SULFUR   A nonmetallic element. Used as a stimulant and to kill parasites. It is employed, particularly in the form of shampoo, in the treatment of skin and scalp diseases.

SUNSCREEN   Chemical in suntan lotions which screens out the sunburning rays, which are from 2,900 to 3,200 Angstrom units, but permits the tanning rays to filter through.

SWEAT   Liquid secreted to the skin surface through the sweat ducts. Eccrine and apocrine glands produce different varieties of sweat.

TERRAMYCIN   An antibiotic, effective in treatment of skin infections.

THIOGLYCOLATE   Organic sulfur compound used as a depilatory and in hair-waving solutions.

THROMBOPHLEBITIS   Inflammation of the veins which very frequently occurs when one is taking the birth-control Pill.

TINEA   See RINGWORM.

TRACTION ALOPECIA   Loss of hair due to continuous traction, as by wearing hair in a ponytail or using rollers overnight.

ULCER, SKIN   A depressed area of the skin due to loss or death of the skin's superficial layers; associated with infection or impaired blood circulation.

ULTRAVIOLET LIGHT   A range of invisible radiation consisting of short wavelengths that produce tanning of the skin. Used in diagnosis of ringworm infections of the scalp.

URTICARIA   Allergic reaction of the skin; hives. May be acute or chronic.

VACCINE   Medicinal biological preparation, usually containing killed organisms, which is used to produce or increase immunity.

VENEREAL DISEASE   Genital infection transmitted by a germ during sexual intercourse.

VERRUCA   A small tumor on the skin, usually hard; wart. Caused by virus.

VESICLE   Sharply circumscribed accumulation of free fluid; blister.

VIRUS   A submicroscopic agent that causes diseases. Considered a living organism; passes through filters that stop the passage of bacteria.

VITAMINS   A group of organic substances present in food, or synthetic in origin, which are essential to normal health. Their lack results in deficiency diseases.

VITILIGO   Presence of white areas on the skin due to sudden loss of pigment. Occurs without previous inflammation.

INDEX

abrasion, 11, 46, 96
abstinence, 184–185
Achilles tendon, 135
acid mantle, 5, 19
acne, 5, 6–15, 81, 188–189
  causes of, 7–9, 188
  control of, 10–14
  cystic, 9
  diet and, 9, 13
  hormones and, 7–8, 81
  in males *vs.* females, 6, 8
  scarring from, 13, 14–15, 196–197
  statistics on, 6
  sweat, 9, 13
  treatment of, 10–15, 179, 189
ACTH, 26
adrenal glands, 90, 94
aerobic system, 134
aftershaves, 18, 29, 59
Al-Anon, 173
Alateen, 173
albinos, 4
alcohol, 156, 166–173
  abuse of, 171–173, 188–189
  brain affected by, 168
  driving and, 167, 171–172
  as food, 166
  other drugs combined with, 167, 172

physical reaction to, 167–169
quiz on, 170
Alcoholics Anonymous, 173
alcohol-saturated pads, 17–18
allergens:
  in cosmetic preparations, 60–61
  kinds of, 23
allergies, 23–30, 188–189
  contact, 23, 24–28, 188
  cosmetics and, 21, 26–27, 59–62
  defined, 23
  food, 23–24, 188
  hair dyes and, 26, 101–103, 107
  inhalants and, 23, 24, 188
"alligator skin," 37
alopecia:
  areata, totalis, and universalis, 85–87
  from diseases and infections, 85, 90–91
  after pregnancy, 85
  seborrheic, 85, 90
  traction, 87
  see also baldness
American Medical Association (AMA), 147
amphetamines, 157, 165
Amytal, 165
anaerobic system, 134, 136, 139
anemia, 86

215

ABOUT THE AUTHORS

Dr. Irwin I. Lubowe is Clinical Professor of Dermatology at the New York Medical College–Metropolitan Hospital Center in New York City and Chief Dermatologist at the Metropolitan Hospital Clinic. A practicing specialist noted for his research work on the care, hygiene and treatment of the skin and hair, Dr. Lubowe has contributed many scientific articles on these subjects to medical and technical journals. His highly praised books include *New Hope for Your Hair* and *New Hope for Your Skin.* His home is in New York City.

Barbara Huss (Mrs. Reeve Limeburner) is a writer who specializes in the subjects of grooming, health and good looks for young adults. A former editor of *American Girl,* she has conducted good grooming and fashion shows in leading stores throughout the country, and has also appeared on radio and television. In addition, she has written extensively on cosmetics and drugs for leading New York advertising agencies and a worldwide pharmaceutical firm. She now writes and lives in Old Lyme, Connecticut.